A Special Issue of
The European Journal of Cognitive Psychology

Neuroimaging of Mental Imagery

Edited by

Michel Denis
Université de Paris-Sud, Orsay, France

Emmanuel Mellet
Université de Caen and Université Rene-Descartes, France

and

Stephen M. Kosslyn
Harvard University and Massachusetts General Hospital, MA, USA

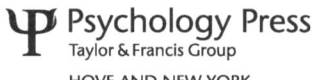

Psychology Press
Taylor & Francis Group
HOVE AND NEW YORK

Published in 2004
by Psychology Press Ltd
27 Church Road, Hove, East Sussex BN3 2FA

Simultaneously published in the USA and Canada
by Psychology Press
711 Third Avenue, New York, NY 10017

First issued in paperback 2015

*Psychology Press is an imprint of the Taylor & Francis Group,
an informa business*

British Library Cataloguing in Publication Data
A catalogue record for this book is available from the British Library

ISBN 13: 978-1-138-87802-0 (pbk)
ISBN 13: 978-1-8416-9973-8 (hbk)

ISSN 0954–1446

Cover design by Hybert Design, Waltham St Lawrence, Berkshire, UK
Typeset by DP Photosetting, Aylesbury, Buckinghamshire, UK

Contents*

---

*This book is also a special issue of the *European Journal of Cognitive
Psychology* and forms Issue 5 of Volume 16 (2004).

EUROPEAN JOURNAL OF COGNITIVE PSYCHOLOGY, 2004, *16* (5), 625–630

Neuroimaging of mental imagery: An introduction

Michel Denis

*Groupe Cognition Humaine, LIMSI-CNRS, Université de Paris-Sud,
Orsay, France*

Emmanuel Mellet

*Groupe d'Imagerie Neurofonctionnelle, Université de Caen, and
Université René-Descartes, France*

Stephen M. Kosslyn

*Department of Psychology, Harvard University, Cambridge, and Department of
Neurology, Massachusetts General Hospital, Boston, MA, USA*

Since the earliest days of scientific psychology, the value of mental imagery in comprehension, memory, and reasoning has been recognised and studied. The massive amount of data collected in this domain of research has revealed that the human mind is often inclined toward the most direct contact possible with the objects of its focus, using mental images in addition to and sometimes instead of indirect or more remote contact based on symbolic, language-like representational systems. In scientific thinking, as in every other form of thinking, imagery is considered an irreplaceable tool, which efficiently supplements more abstract forms of reasoning (Denis, Logie, Cornoldi, de Vega, & Engelkamp, 2001; Shepard, 1988).

This issue of the *European Journal of Cognitive Psychology* addresses this traditional topic in psychology, but does so in a new way—using neuroimaging. It is not surprising that cognitive science has increasingly relied on methods that provide data about the neural substrates of cognition, in particular derived from

Correspondence should be addressed to Michel Denis, Groupe Cognition Humaine, LIMSI-CNRS, Université de Paris-Sud, BP 133, 91403 Orsay Cedex, France. Email: denis@limsi.fr

The papers that were submitted for publication in the present special issue were reviewed in accordance with the standard peer-review procedure. The invited co-editors would like to express their appreciation to the referees who provided expertise and advice during the reviewing process: Giorgio Ganis, Olivier Houdé, Alumit Ishai, Fred Mast, Bernard Mazoyer, Mauro Pesenti, Laurent Petit, Viviane Pouthas, John T. E. Richardson, William L. Thompson, Nathalie Tzourio-Mazoyer, Annalena Venneri, Mark E. Wheeler, and Jeff Zacks. They are also grateful to Kate Moysen, from Psychology Press, for her dedication to the project, her professional support, and her patience throughout the production process of this special issue.

http://www.tandf.co.uk/journals/pp/09541446.html   DOI:10.1080/09541440440000096 neuroimaging methods. And the study of mental imagery was among the first cognitive domains that inspired significant amounts of neuroimaging research. Two decades after the publication of Roland and Friberg's (1985) pioneering work on the variations of cerebral blood flow that accompany the visualisation of a familiar route, mental imagery is still the focus of a large amount of neuroimaging research. The questions being asked by cognitive scientists are easy to formulate—but the answers sometimes may be difficult to obtain. For example: Does mental imagery share common cortical structures with those known to be active during perception and motor control? How do differences in brain activation inform us about the nature of different types of imagery? How do differences in brain activation inform us about the different strategies people can adopt when using imagery? What do the temporal relations among activations of different brain areas tell us about the course of information processing? How do individual differences in the degree of activation produce individual differences in performance?

These are the types of questions that the contributors to the present special issue of the journal have asked, and have begun to answer in detail in a series of original neuroimaging studies. These studies rely on positron emission tomography (PET) and functional magnetic resonance imaging (fMRI). These techniques are used in the context of a variety of cognitive tasks involving memory, problem solving, and other processes. A strong emphasis is placed on individual differences, which have long been recognized as requiring special attention in order to provide comprehensive accounts of the results of imagery experiments.

Today, we are far beyond the time when cerebral specialisation was conceived only in terms of hemispheric differences. Not only are cerebral regions now carefully differentiated in terms of their functional specialisation, but also imagery tasks are contrasted in terms of their specific requirements (such as representing shape versus spatial relations). Neurofunctional studies of imagery have demonstrated that the activation patterns during imagery depend strongly on the tasks performed (e.g., Thompson & Kosslyn, 2000). One of the merits of the neuroimaging approach to studying mental imagery is that it focuses us on fine-grained analyses of the processes required to perform specific tasks—which leads us to draw distinctions among what previously were lumped together under the general label of ''imagery tasks''.

There is a consensus that retrieving visual representations from memory involves some form of reactivation of the cortical structures that were activated when these representations initially were encoded. In the first paper of the present issue, Todd Handy and his colleagues attempt to establish whether brain activity differs in two circumstances, when a person visualises an object by recalling a recently encoded picture of that object versus when a person visualises an object by retrieving visual information about the object stored in long-term memory. In other words, the aim of this research is to discover whether the activating processes responsible for imagery are affected by the particular strategy one employs. The data collected in a blocked fMRI design show that the left ventral cortex in the fusiform gyrus is activated in both conditions, whereas the frontal cortex is activated differently in the two conditions—which suggests that partly different mechanisms underlie the two retrieval strategies. In addition to apparent differences in the two retrieval mechanisms, the results speak in favour of a common network in the left hemisphere that is activated in both cases.

The next paper summarises studies that explore the neural correlates of a spatial imagery task. A nice feature of neuroimaging studies is that they provide an opportunity to revisit classic imagery paradigms. Here, Luigi Trojano and his colleagues recorded fMRI measures while participants compared mentally the angles formed by the two hands of a clock, an adaptation of the "mental clocks" task originally designed by Allan Paivio (1978). The results of the studies document the role of the cortical areas in the posterior parietal cortex in spatial mental imagery, even in the absence of any visual stimulation. Furthermore, the comparison of tasks involving the categorical and coordinate processing of spatial mental images reveals that both types of processing share a common region of activation in the superior parietal lobule, but that the two sorts of processing are not identical. Another interesting finding bears on an issue that has elicited much controversy during the past decade, namely the circumstances in which imagery induces activation in early visual areas—especially in cases where abstract or schematic patterns are imagined, without requiring the inspection of fine-grained visuospatial representations.

This controversy is directly addressed in the following paper. Taking advantage of a database of nine PET experiments conducted in their laboratory, Angélique Mazard and her colleagues directly compare spatial and object imagery tasks, with the aim of discovering which brain areas are activated in common and which are not. Their meta-analysis reveals both common and distinct areas that are activated during the two sorts of imagery. In some respects, the most illuminating result concerns a crucial difference during spatial versus object imagery: These researchers report that spatial imagery activates the superior part of the parietal cortex, whereas object imagery engages the anterior part of the ventral pathway. More specifically, the early visual cortex tends to be activated by object imagery, while it is deactivated by spatial imagery. This analysis strongly suggests that the early visual cortex plays a role in the visualisation of figural information, although large interindividual variations are also evident in the activity of this region. Thus, this meta-analysis contributes to the ongoing debate about the role of early visual areas in visual mental imagery (e.g., Roland & Gulyas, 1994).

A further attempt to delineate the subprocesses serving imagery is found in the experiment reported by Stephen Kosslyn and his colleagues. They used PET to monitor brain activity while participants performed four tasks: forming high-resolution images, generating images from distinct segments, inspecting images to parse them, and rotating images. The innovative feature of this study is that rather than compare a test condition to a baseline, as is the convention in neuroimaging research, these researchers rely on multiple regression analyses. In these analyses, variations in response times and error rates are regressed onto variations in regional cerebral blood flow, with the goal of discovering in which areas variations in blood flow predict variations in performance. This method is an alternative to the subtractive method, in that it does not inform us about the brain areas that underlie performance, but rather about those regions that underlie *variations* in performance in specific tasks. The results revealed not only that different areas predict performance in different tasks, but also that the number of brain areas that predicts performance lines up with the complexity of the tasks.

Other challenging issues are introduced in the following three papers. Mental rotation and the meaning of parietal activation in functional neuroimaging are the subjects of Vinoth Jagaroo's theory-driven review. The discussion is grounded in the widely recognised fact that the posterior parietal cortex is activated during mental rotation. This activation may be interpreted as reflecting a specialised parietal function that underlies the transformational process itself, or this activation could reflect the role of the parietal lobe in directing eye movements. By highlighting the centrality of coordinate transformations in the process under study, the author suggests some interesting lines of future work on functional imaging of mental rotation.

The next paper addresses the issue of sensory integration and intermodal differences. The neuroimaging literature has focused on visual imagery and the question of shared mechanisms for visual perception and visual imagery. This study by Marta Olivetti Belardinelli and her colleagues used fMRI to record brain activation while participants generated images in eight modalities (visual, auditory, tactile, olfactory, gustatory, kinaesthetic, visceral, and abstract). The newest piece of information reported here is that the posterior portion of the middle-inferior temporal cortex is recruited by all imagery modalities, indicating that this region is not specific to visual imagery, as previously assumed by the authors of studies that focused solely on visual imagery. Parietal and prefrontal areas show a more heterogeneous pattern of activation for the modalities considered. The data converge on the idea that the generation of images involves high-level processes that are independent of modality-specific representations.

The final contribution to this special issue reports one of the first attempts to collect PET data in people engaged in a high-level type of problem solving, namely, chess playing. By examining the brains of experts during blindfold chess, it is possible to access the neural representations of mental images constructed during this very complex task. Pertti Saariluoma and his colleagues compared performance in a memory task (which requires spatial information storage) and problem solving (which in addition calls for access to long-term memory and planning) in experienced chess players, using their performance in an attention task as a baseline. The findings clearly show that the pattern of brain activation is different in these two tasks. In particular, the memory task activates the temporal areas, whereas problem solving activates several frontal areas. This research opens the door to the speculation that experts' chess-specific images may not necessarily be represented in the brain in the same way as ordinary mental images.

The explosion of interest in neuroimaging methods among researchers who study cognition cannot be explained solely by the appeal of seeing pretty pictures of brain activity. Rather, these sophisticated methods force scientists to relate theories of mental processing to the brain itself, and invite scientists to develop detailed models of cognition that do more than explain behaviour—that also specify the underlying mechanisms in biologically plausible terms. Cognitive scientists, and in particular those who focus on the study of mental imagery, have no excuse for ignoring the value of these techniques. But the techniques are not a "magic bullet". They are only useful if combined with clearly focused questions that are rooted in theoretical issues. Moreover, researchers must take care not to fall into the trap of assuming that the pretty coloured pictures provided by today's impressive machines are the direct reflections of *mental images*, but instead must keep in mind that they are viewing evidence of underlying *neuronal activity*—which is not the same thing as a mental representation, let alone the experience that a type of representation may evoke. The challenge is to use this information to build theoretical models of the cognitive processes that are supported by cerebral activations.

Consistent with a general trend in the papers published in psychology journals, the reader will notice that the lists of co-authors of the published papers tend to be increasingly long. This reflects the fact that neuroimaging is a highly collaborative and interdisciplinary domain. This trend probably also suggests that some disciplinary borders will soon have to be reconsidered in the field of human cognition. Needless to say, this collaborative endeavour goes along with extensive international cooperation, which is reflected here by the fact that the seven papers involve authors from a total of eight different countries.

The present special issue of the *European Journal of Cognitive Psychology* is an outgrowth of the Eighth European Workshop on Imagery and Cognition (EWIC), which was organised in Saint-Malo, France, in April 2001, by Michel Denis and Maryvonne Carfantan. Since the launching of the EWIC meetings in 1986, the presence of neuroimaging methods in research on mental imagery has steadily increased. The 2001 edition of EWIC included a special session on Neuroimaging Investigations of Mental Imagery, whose content served as a starting point for shaping this special issue of the *European Journal of Cognitive Psychology* on the neuroimaging of mental imagery. A call for papers was widely circulated. Some of the original papers presented at the workshop were published elsewhere, while newly submitted papers were accepted, thus forming a set of seven original papers. The invited co-editors appreciated very much the enthusiastic response of Claus Bundesen, Editor, to their proposal of devoting a full special issue to neuroimaging investigations of this major topic within cognitive psychology. We hope that this special issue will be a source of inspiration for further research on a fascinating facet of human cognition.

PrEview proof published online June 2004

REFERENCES

Denis, M., Logie, R. H., Cornoldi, C., de Vega, M., & Engelkamp, J. (Eds.). (2001). *Imagery, language, and visuo-spatial thinking.* Hove, UK: Psychology Press.

Paivio, A. (1978). Comparisons of mental clocks. *Journal of Experimental Psychology: Human Perception and Performance, 4,* 61–71.

Roland, P. E., & Friberg, L. (1985). Localization of cortical areas activated by thinking. *Journal of Neurophysiology, 53,* 1219–1243.

Roland, P. E., & Gulyas, B. (1994). Visual imagery and visual representation. *Trends in Neurosciences, 17,* 281–287.

Shepard, R. N. (1988). The imagination of the scientist. In K. Egan & D. Nadaner (Eds.), *Imagination and education* (pp. 153–185). New York: Teachers College Press.

Thompson, W. L., & Kosslyn, S. M. (2000). Neural systems activated during visual mental imagery: A review and meta-analyses. In A. W. Toga & J. C. Mazziotta (Eds.), *Brain mapping: The systems* (pp. 535–560). San Diego, CA: Academic Press.

EUROPEAN JOURNAL OF COGNITIVE PSYCHOLOGY, 2004, *16* (5), 631–652

Visual imagery and memory: Do retrieval strategies affect what the mind's eye sees?

Todd C. Handy

Department of Psychology, University of British Columbia, Vancouver, BC, Canada

Michael B. Miller

Center for Cognitive Neuroscience, Dartmouth College, Hanover, NH, and Department of Psychology, University of California, Santa Barbara, CA, USA

Bjoern Schott

Department of Neurology II, University of Magdeburg, Germany

Neha M. Shroff and Petr Janata

Center for Cognitive Neuroscience, and Department of Psychological and Brain Sciences, Dartmouth College, Hanover, NH, USA

John D. Van Horn, Souheil Inati, and Scott T. Grafton

Center for Cognitive Neuroscience, Department of Psychological and Brain Sciences, and Dartmouth Brain Imaging Center, Dartmouth College, Hanover, NH, USA

Michael S. Gazzaniga

Center for Cognitive Neuroscience, and Department of Psychological and Brain Sciences, Dartmouth College, Hanover, NH, USA

A variety of visual mental imagery tasks have been shown to activate regions of visual cortex that subserve the perception of visual events. Here fMRI was used to examine whether imagery-related visuocortical activity is modulated if imagery content is held constant but there is a change in the memory retrieval strategy used to invoke imagery. Participants were scanned while visualising common objects in two different conditions: (a) recalling recently encoded pictures and (b) based on

Correspondence should be addressed to Todd C. Handy, Department of Psychology, University of British Columbia, 2136 West Mall, Vancouver, BC, V6T 1Z4, Canada. Email: tchandy@psych.ubc.ca

This research was funded by NIH grant NS17778-21 awarded to MSG, and the Dartmouth Brain Imaging Center. We thank Bill Kelley, Andy Yonelinas, and Emrah Düzel for helpful comments, and Tammy Laroche for her assistance with data collection.

© 2004 Psychology Press Ltd
http://www.tandf.co.uk/journals/pp/09541446.html   DOI: 10.1080/09541440340000457

their knowledge of concrete nouns. Results showed that retrieval-related activations in frontal cortex were bilateral when pictures were visualised but left-lateralised when nouns were visualised. In posterior brain regions, both imagery conditions led to activation in the same set of circumscribed areas in left temporal-parietal cortex, including a region of the left fusiform gyrus that has previously been implicated in visual imagery. These findings suggest that the posterior network activated during imagery did not vary with strategic task-related changes in the frontal network used to retrieve imagery content from memory.

Retrieving information from memory allows us to visualise places and things not currently available in our perceptual milieu. Over the last decade it has become increasingly clear that the neural basis of visual mental imagery is tied to the endogenous activation of cortical areas subserving visual perception (e.g., Behrmann, 2000; Denis, Goncalves, & Memmi, 1995; Farah, 1995; Kosslyn, Ganis, & Thompson, 2001; Mellet, Petit, Mazoyer, Denis, & Tzourio, 1998a; Roland & Gulyás, 1994; Sakai & Miyashita, 1993). The emerging consensus is that the retrieval of visual representations from memory leads to the reactivation of cortical areas that were initially activated during the perceptual encoding of those representations (e.g., Ishai & Sagi, 1997; Ishai, Ungerleider, & Haxby, 2000; Kosslyn, Thompson, & Alpert, 1997; Krelman, Koch, & Fried, 2000). In support of this ''reactivation'' hypothesis, visual imagery generation has been shown to increase activity in both primary visual cortex (e.g., Kosslyn et al., 1993, 1999; Kosslyn, Thompson, Kim, & Alpert, 1995b; Le Bihan, Turner, Zeffiro, Cuénod, Jezzard, & Bonnerot, 1993; Thompson, Kosslyn, Sukel, & Alpert, 2001) and object recognition areas of ventral temporal cortex (e.g., D'Esposito et al., 1997; Fletcher, Frith, Grasby, Shallice, Frackowiak, & Dolan, 1995; Ishai et al., 2000; Mellet, Tzourio, Denis, & Mazoyer, 1998b; O'Craven & Kanwisher, 2000; Wheeler, Petersen, & Buckner, 2000). Integral to this cortical reactivation is the retrieval of imagery content from memory. Nevertheless, the question of how—or even if—strategic memory retrieval processes influence reactivation during imagery has received comparatively little attention.

The issue centres on appreciating the different ways in which the content of visual imagery can be generated from memory, and how this may alter the strategic retrieval processes invoked. In one commonly used paradigm, participants are first presented with a set of objects to encode as memoranda, and then cued to visually recall the items that have been encoded (e.g., Kosslyn et al., 1995b, 1999; Le Bihan et al., 1993; Thompson et al., 2001; Wheeler et al., 2000). A second common paradigm has relied on more general or semantic-based knowledge for imagery generation, where participants are simply given the names of common visual objects as the cues for imagery (e.g., D'Esposito et al., 1997; Mellet et al., 1998b). Although both paradigms may give rise to vivid imagery in the mind's eye, the paradigms may also lead to nontrivial differences in the strategic processes engaged during the retrieval of imagery content from memory.

In particular, studies of memory retrieval have shown that activation of right frontal cortex (RFC) appears to vary in a systematic fashion with the parameters of the retrieval task involved (for a review, see Buckner & Wheeler, 2001). In this regard, the collective evidence predicts that recalling the visual appearance of objects encoded as temporally unique (or episodic) events should engage strategic processes in RFC, but that RFC activation should be reduced or absent when visualising the appearance of common objects in more semantic-type retrieval tasks that place no emphasis on when or where imagery content has been acquired (e.g., Buckner, Raichle, Miezin, & Petersen, 1996; Cabeza, Kapur, Craik, McIntosh, Houle, & Tulving, 1997; Düzel et al., 1999; Fletcher et al., 1995; Gabrieli et al., 1996; Haxby, Ungerleider, Horwitz, Maisog, Rapoport, & Grady, 1996; Nyberg, Habib, McIntosh, & Tulving, 2000; Schacter, Alpert, Savage, Rauch, & Albert, 1996; Tulving, Kapur, Craik, Moscovitch, & Houle, 1994; Wagner, Poldrack, Eldridge, Desmond, Glover, & Gabrieli, 1998). Although debate exists over how to functionally interpret task-related differences in RFC activation during retrieval (e.g., Buckner & Wheeler, 2001; Kelley, Buckner, & Petersen, 1998; Nyberg, Cabeza, & Tulving, 1998), the issue is tangential to the goal here. Stated simply, if the aforementioned predictions are correct, does the engagement of retrieval processes in RFC influence the extent to which visual imagery reactivates visual cortex, relative to imagery conditions showing less reliance on strategic processing in RFC?

The question sits at a key juncture in the links between imagery and memory. A recent meta-analysis of neuroimaging studies has suggested that medial occipital cortex (MOC) and bilateral occipitotemporal cortex are all regions labile to activation during imagery, but that there is unexplained variance in how these regions have responded to task conditions across studies (Thompson & Kosslyn, 2000). The growing belief is that the content of imagery plays a critical role in determining visuocortical activation during imagery, with MOC involvement more likely when high resolution images are necessary for optimal task performance (e.g., Kosslyn et al., 2001; Mellet et al., 1998a). Indeed, behavioural reports have suggested that imagery predicated on semantic memories may be less vivid or detailed than imagery generated from event-specific, episodic memories (e.g., Brewer & Pani, 1996). Such evidence suggests that the source of a visual mental image in memory may be sufficient to influence the content or resolution of imagery, altering in turn the pattern of imagery-related activity in visual cortex. Consistent with this possibility, recent neuroimaging evidence has indicated that image resolution alone may not determine whether MOC activity will be invoked during imagery (Thompson et al., 2001).

Taking a key first step in understanding how strategic memory processes may influence imagery-related cortical reactivation, Mellet et al. (2000) recently examined how the strategy used at the time of encoding affects the pattern of imagery-related activation in posterior cortical areas. The same participant cohort was scanned using positron emission tomography (PET) while a set of objects was imaged that (1) had been viewed during encoding, or (2) that had been verbally described at encoding with no accompanying visual object representation. Results showed that the form of encoding—visual or verbal based—did not affect the network of areas in posterior cortex activated during imagery. Methodologically, the study is notable in that the content of imagery was held constant between conditions while memory processing associated with imagery content was varied. Switching the focus from encoding to retrieval, our aim was to examine the effect of different retrieval strategies on cortical reactivation during imagery.

Specifically, we manipulated within-subjects the retrieval conditions under which visual imagery was generated while participants were scanned in a blocked fMRI design. There were three experimental conditions, as summarised in Figure 1. In the first condition participants were auditorily cued to visualise objects that were encoded just prior to the scanning run (pictures imagery condition). In the second condition participants were auditorily cued to visualise the appearance of concrete nouns that were common visual objects (nouns imagery condition). As a third condition participants were also scanned while encoding the object memoranda for the pictures condition (visual encoding condition). The paradigm thus held constant the participant cohort and the qualitative content of imagery while varying the nature of the task used to retrieve imagery content. Data analysis then centred on determining whether (1) there were differences in anterior cortical regions activated between the two imagery tasks, and (2) whether imagery-related reactivation of visual cortex co-varied with the imagery condition.

METHODS

Participants

Fifteen healthy, right-handed adults participated in the experiment (10 female, 18–29 years of age). All had normal or corrected-to-normal vision and gave their informed written consent prior to scanning. All methods and procedures were approved by the Dartmouth College Committee for the Protection of Human Subjects.

Procedure and apparatus

Each participant was scanned under two different imagery conditions. In the pictures condition, participants were cued to recall visual images of pictures they had just encoded (see below). In the nouns condition, participants were cued to recall the appearance of various common objects—explicit instructions were

EPOCHS

CONDITION	TASK	REST
ENCODING:	Eyes open. Viewing objects. Hearing object name.	Eyes open. Viewing blank screen. Hearing abstract word.
PICTURES:	Eyes closed. Imaging encoded object. Hearing object name.	Eyes closed. No imagery. Hearing abstract word.
NOUNS:	Eyes closed. Imaging object noun. Hearing object name.	Eyes closed. No imagery. Hearing abstract word.

Figure 1. Task conditions. In the encoding condition participants were presented with the objects used as memoranda for imagery generation in the pictures condition. In the nouns condition imagery was based on hearing concrete nouns that named common visual objects. Participants listened to abstract words during all rest epochs, and the two imagery conditions (pictures and nouns) were performed with eyes closed for the duration of the functional run.

given that images should be based on a general understanding of how the named object appears rather than in reference to a specific event associated with the named object. Both imagery conditions were performed with eyes closed in a darkened scanning room, and single words naming each object were presented over headphones as the cues for imagery. Auditory stimulation was controlled using VAPP stimulus presentation software (http://nilab.psychiatry.ubc.ca/vapp/) running on a Dell Pentium PC and amplified via stereo receiver (Technics S4-EX10). The stimulus signal was passed through an electric-acoustic audio signal transducer (Etymotic Research, ER-30 transducer) and presented to the participant via rubber tubing mounted into the headphones and equipped with 3 mm foam eartips (Etymotic Research) for insertion into the ear canal.

Participants performed two functional runs in each of the two imagery conditions. Each run consisted of 38 s epochs of "imagery" that were interleaved with 30 s epochs of "rest". In order to keep auditory stimulation operationally equivalent across all epoch types, during rest epochs participants passively listened to abstract words (e.g., "unity" and "belief") presented over the headphones at the same temporal rate as in the imagery epochs. Within each imagery epoch 10 imagery cues were given, one every 3.5 s, with an additional 3 s blank interval at the end of the epoch; within each rest epoch eight abstract words were given, one every 3.5 s, with an additional 2 s blank interval at the end of the epoch. Each functional run began with a rest epoch followed by a task epoch, a pattern that repeated three more times for a total of four epochs of each type within each functional run. In order to minimise confusion as to whether a to-be-imaged object had been encoded or not, the pictures and nouns conditions were presented in separate functional runs, with the order of runs counterbalanced between subjects. In all four functional runs the difference between rest and imagery epochs was emphasised by using a female voice during imagery epochs and a male voice during rest epochs.

In order to provide the memoranda for the pictures condition, each run in this condition was preceded by a functional run during which the to-be-encoded pictures were presented (encoding condition). In each encoding run colour pictures of common objects (e.g., a flower, a helicopter, a shovel) were rear-projected (Epson ELP-7000 LCD projector) onto a screen at the participant's feet using the stimulus presentation software described above. Participants viewed the screen using a headcoil-mounted mirror. Each picture was presented for 2 s, against a white background, followed by a 1.5 s blank interval when only a fixation point was present. In conjunction with each picture, the participants heard the name of the object over headphones, the word that would then serve as the imagery cue during the subsequent pictures run. During rest epochs participants maintained fixation on a grey screen while listening to abstract words. In order to facilitate comparison between visual areas active during visual perception and visual imagery, the timing and auditory aspects of the task and rest epochs were identical to those used in the two imagery conditions described above. At the beginning of each encoding run participants were informed that they would be asked to later recall images of the pictures presented. The order of recall in the pictures condition that followed was randomised relative to the order of visual presentation during the encoding condition.

A total of 80 different colour images were used for the encoding condition, 40 in each of the two functional runs. As a result, in the pictures condition each of these encoded pictures was imaged exactly once. Likewise, there were 80 different nouns used in the nouns condition (40 in each functional run), with no overlap between this set of items and the set of 80 items used in the pictures and encoding conditions. Because each of the two functional runs in the pictures condition was immediately preceded by the paired encoding functional run (see above), the delay between the encoding and subsequent imagery of each picture was approximately 6–8 min, on average. The items used for imagery in both imagery conditions were common objects that one might typically encounter in everyday life (e.g., ladder, airplane, doughnut, spoon). As such, items imaged in the pictures and nouns conditions came from a variety of different object categories (e.g., food, tools).

Participants did not manually signal item-by-item success in generating imagery. Instead, they were instructed to closely monitor their rate of imagery failure during each imagery run. The first 10 participants in the study were asked to report at the end of each imagery run whether they had had more than five failed imagery attempts on that run. Nine participants reported a negative response to this question on every run; one participant reported no imagery on any run and was excluded from subsequent analysis. To more precisely quantify imagery failure, the final five participants reported at the end of each run their best estimate of how many failed imagery attempts had occurred on that run.

fMRI acquisition and analysis

Data were collected using a 1.5T SIGNA scanner (GE Medical Systems) with a fast gradient system for echo-planar imaging (EPI). Foam padding was used for head stabilisation. EPI images sensitive to the blood oxygen-level-dependent (BOLD) signal were acquired using a gradient-echo pulse sequence (TR = 2000 ms, TE = 35 ms, flip angle = 90°, 27 contiguous slices at 5 mm thick, and an in-plane resolution of 64 × 64 pixels in a FOV of 24 cm, producing voxels of 3.75 mm × 3.75 mm × 5 mm). Each scan began with four 2 s "dummy" shots to allow for steady-state tissue magnetisation. High-resolution, T1-weighted axial images were also taken of each subject (TR = 25 ms, TE = 6 ms, bandwidth = 15.6 kHz, voxel size = 0.9375 mm × 1.25 mm × 1.2 mm). Image reconstruction was performed on-line. Off-line data were processed and analysed using SPM99 (http://www.fil.ion.ucl.ac.uk/spm). For each subject the EPI images were corrected for motion (Friston, Williams, Howard, Frackowiak, & Turner, 1996), the EPI and anatomical images were co-registered and then spatially normalised into stereotaxic coordinates approximating the atlas of Talairach and Tournoux (1988) (Friston, Holmes, Worsley, Poline, Frith, & Frackowiak, 1995b). Finally, the normalised EPI images were spatially smoothed using an isotropic 8 mm Gaussian kernel.

Single-subject statistical analysis was based on a multiple regression using the general linear model (Friston, Ashburner, Frith, Poline, Heather, & Frackowiak, 1995a). Prior to parameter estimation the time series data for each subject were proportionally scaled in order to remove global changes in the BOLD signal intensity (but see Aguirre, Zarahn, & D'Esposito, 1998; Desjardins, Kiehl, & Liddle, 2001). Imagery and encoding epochs were modelled using a box-car reference waveform that was convolved with the haemodynamic response function (HRF). Voxel-wise mean parameter estimates (ßs) were then calculated within each run in order to quantify the degree to which the BOLD signal approximated the convolved HRF reference waveform; linear, quadratic, and cubic regressors were included in the regression model as effects of non-interest. Subsequent group-level analyses were based on a random-effects model using one-sample t-tests.

RESULTS

Behavioural performance

Participants were required to monitor and report their rate of imagery failure during each functional run (see Methods). For participants reporting the specific number of imagery failures per run, the mean in the pictures condition was 3.4 failed attempts per run (range: 0–8) and the mean in the nouns condition was 2.6 failed attempts per run (range: 0–5). Upon debriefing at the conclusion of the experiment, all 14 participants included in the data set reported vivid mental imagery during the imagery epochs.

fMRI data

Region of interest criteria.   Analysis of fMRI data focused on two primary questions. First, was there evidence that different retrieval processes were engaged in right prefrontal cortex during the two imagery conditions? Second, did visuocortical activation differ between imagery conditions? In order to address these questions, five contrasts of interest were performed: (1) comparing task to rest epochs in the pictures imagery condition, (2) comparing task to rest epochs in the nouns imagery condition, (3) comparing task to rest epochs in the visual encoding condition, (4) a direct comparison between the pictures and nouns conditions showing areas more active during the pictures condition, and (5) a direct comparison between the pictures and nouns conditions showing areas more active during the nouns condition. In the group analyses all five contrasts were thresholded at a t probability value of $p < .0001$ (uncorrected) with a minimum cluster size of 10 contiguous voxels. At this criterion level no significant voxel clusters were found in the nouns > pictures contrast. The significant clusters in the four remaining contrasts of interest are shown in Figure 2. Talairach coordinates (Talairach & Tournoux, 1988) and statistics for all clusters in anterior and posterior cortical regions are reported in Tables 1 and 2, respectively.

The data in Figure 2 established the initial regions of interest (ROIs). Further analyses were restricted to ROIs that showed a consistent statistical response across the three imagery contrasts of interest. In particular, for a region to be considered more active in the pictures condition relative to the nouns condition there had to be a significant voxel cluster in that region in the pictures and the

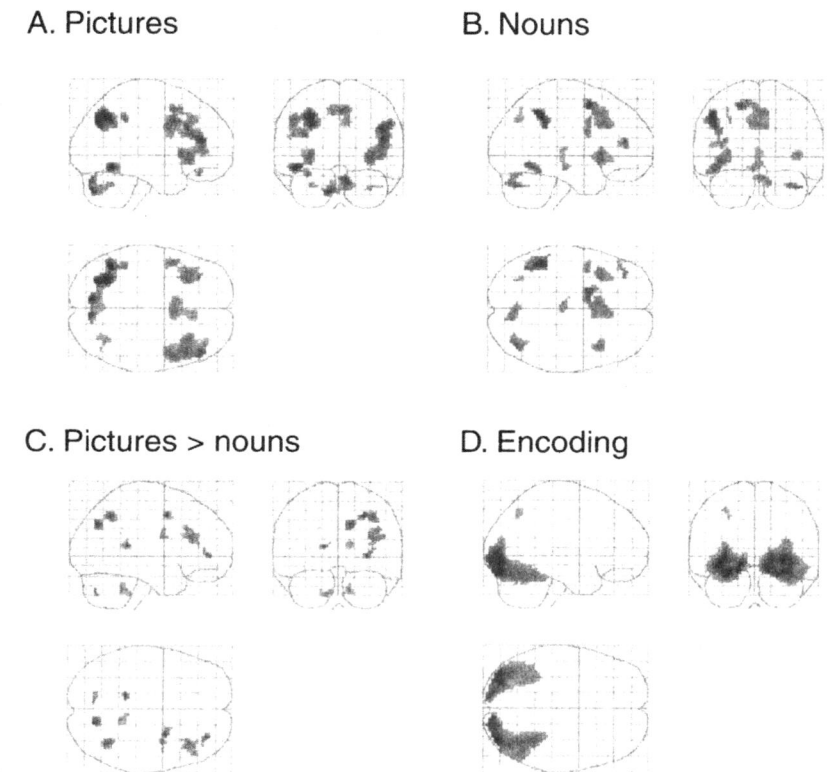

Figure 2.   BOLD response in each contrast of interest. The data shown were thresholded at $p <$ .0001 (uncorrected) with a minimum cluster size of 10 contiguous voxels. These data suggest that the primary differences in the pattern of cortical activation between the pictures **(A)** and nouns **(B)** imagery conditions were in the right frontal and right parietal regions **(C)**. During the visual encoding condition **(D)**, large activations were found in the lateral occipital and ventral temporal regions. At this threshold criterion there were no significant voxel clusters in the nouns > pictures contrast.

pictures > nouns contrast, and no significant voxel cluster in that region in the nouns contrast. For a region to be considered comparably active during both the pictures and nouns conditions there had to be a significant voxel cluster in the region in both the pictures and nouns contrasts, and an absence of a significant voxel cluster in that region in the pictures > nouns contrast. The analyses reported below are restricted to the relevant brain regions meeting these between-contrast criteria. Because the question of memory retrieval processes concerns activations in anterior brain regions and the question of visuocortical activation during imagery concerns responses in posterior brain regions, results are presented in separate subsections based on this anatomical division.

TABLE 1
Significant voxel clusters in anterior cortex as a function of contrast

	Coordinates					Location	
Contrast	x	y	z	k	t	BA	Anatomical label
P_task > P_rest	48	36	18	419	8.42	46/9	R middle frontal gyrus
	−33	36	−21	12	7.73	11	L inferior frontal gyrus
	−48	9	39	84	7.03	47	L middle frontal gyrus
	6	9	48	144	7.02	6	R superior frontal gyrus
	−30	24	0	93	7.19	13	L insula
	−36	27	24	55	6.88	46	L middle frontal gyrus
N_task > N_rest	−18	6	54	271	7.75	6	L medial frontal gyrus
	42	18	3	40	6.91	45	R inferior frontal gyrus
	−36	42	15	26	6.83	46	L middle frontal gyrus
	−39	15	−6	79	6.74	47	L inferior frontal gyrus
	−39	3	27	40	6.05	6	L precentral gyrus
(P_task > P_rest) >	27	3	45	18	8.95	8	R medial frontal gyrus
(N_task > N_rest)	30	45	3	15	8.21	10	R middle frontal gyrus
	36	27	21	59	6.50	45	R inferior frontal gyrus
	36	0	21	16	6.32	13	R insula

Coordinates are in Talairach space, t values are for the statistical maxima within each cluster, the minimum cluster size k was 10 voxels, and all contrasts are reported at $p < .0001$ (uncorrected). P = pictures, N = nouns, BA = Brodmann's area, L = left, R = right.
There were no significant voxel clusters in anterior cortex in the encoding condition.

Anterior activations.   The data shown in Figures 2A and 2B indicate that RFC activation was more pronounced in the pictures condition relative to the nouns condition. The data shown in Figure 2C suggest that all frontal regions significantly more active in the pictures imagery condition relative to the nouns imagery condition were restricted to the right cerebral hemisphere. This conclusion is supported by the data reported in Figure 3, which shows the response of regions in dorsolateral frontal cortex in the three imagery-related contrasts of interest. Significant voxel clusters were found in the right midfrontal gyrus and right insula regions in both the pictures and pictures > nouns contrasts, but not in the nouns contrast. This suggests that activation in these two regions of RFC was restricted to the pictures imagery condition. In comparison, there was a significant voxel cluster in the left precentral gyrus in both the pictures and nouns contrasts, but not the pictures > nouns contrast, suggesting that this region of left prefrontal cortex was comparably active during both imagery conditions.

To quantify the magnitude of response in the ROIs highlighted in Figure 3, for each ROI identified in the group data the mean ß value across all voxels in the cluster was computed within each subject for each of the four contrasts of interest. That is, a single group-level contrast was used to identify an ROI, and

TABLE 2
Significant voxel clusters in posterior cortex as a function of contrast

Contrast	Coordinates					Location	
	x	y	z	k	t	BA	Anatomical label
P_task > P_rest	−30	−69	39	206	10.35	19	L intraparietal sulcus
	−45	−54	−12	66	9.83	37	L fusiform gyrus
	−45	−42	42	24	6.57	40	L inferior parietal lobule
N_task > N_rest	−48	−45	42	78	9.91	40	L inferior parietal lobule
	−42	−54	−12	57	7.19	37	L fusiform gyrus
	−30	−69	39	15	6.07	19	L intraparietal sulcus
(P_task > P_rest) >	15	−72	36	34	8.25	7	R precuneus
(N_task > N_rest)	36	−57	45	39	7.24	40	R inferior parietal lobule
E_task > E_rest	−36	−84	−9	702	16.24	18	L inferior occipital gyrus
	33	−87	0	857	14.58	18	R middle occipital gyrus
	−30	−63	51	17	6.50	7	L superior parietal lobule

Coordinates are in Talairach space, *t* values are for the statistical maxima within each cluster, the minimum cluster size *k* was 10 voxels, and all contrasts are reported at $p < .0001$ (uncorrected). P = pictures, N = nouns, BA = Brodmann's area, L = left, R = right.

then the magnitude of response (ß) in that ROI was computed for each contrast of interest, as shown in the graphs to the right of each brain slice in Figure 3. As a result, the response of an ROI defined in one contrast could be examined in turn in all contrasts of interest. While the clusters reported in the right midfrontal gyrus and right insula region showed evidence of a larger magnitude of response in the pictures imagery condition (Figures 3A and 3C), the clusters reported in the left precentral gyrus manifest a comparable magnitude of response between the two imagery conditions (Figures 3A and 3B). In sum, the data are suggestive of significantly greater activation in RFC during the pictures relative to nouns imagery conditions.

Posterior activations. The only region of visual cortex that was activated during imagery was in the left ventral cortex in the fusiform gyrus. As shown in Figure 4, the same region of the left fusiform gyrus was activated in both the pictures (Figure 4A) and nouns (Figure 4B) imagery conditions. This interpretation was supported by two lines of evidence. First, of the 66 voxels in the pictures cluster and the 57 voxels in the nouns cluster (see Table 2), 42 voxels were common to both voxel clusters. Second, as shown in the graphs in Figure 4A and 4B, each of the two clusters showed a comparable magnitude of response in the two imagery conditions when the mean ß value was computed for each cluster across all contrasts of interests. Importantly, these graphs also indicate that there was a large response in each fusiform ROI during the visual

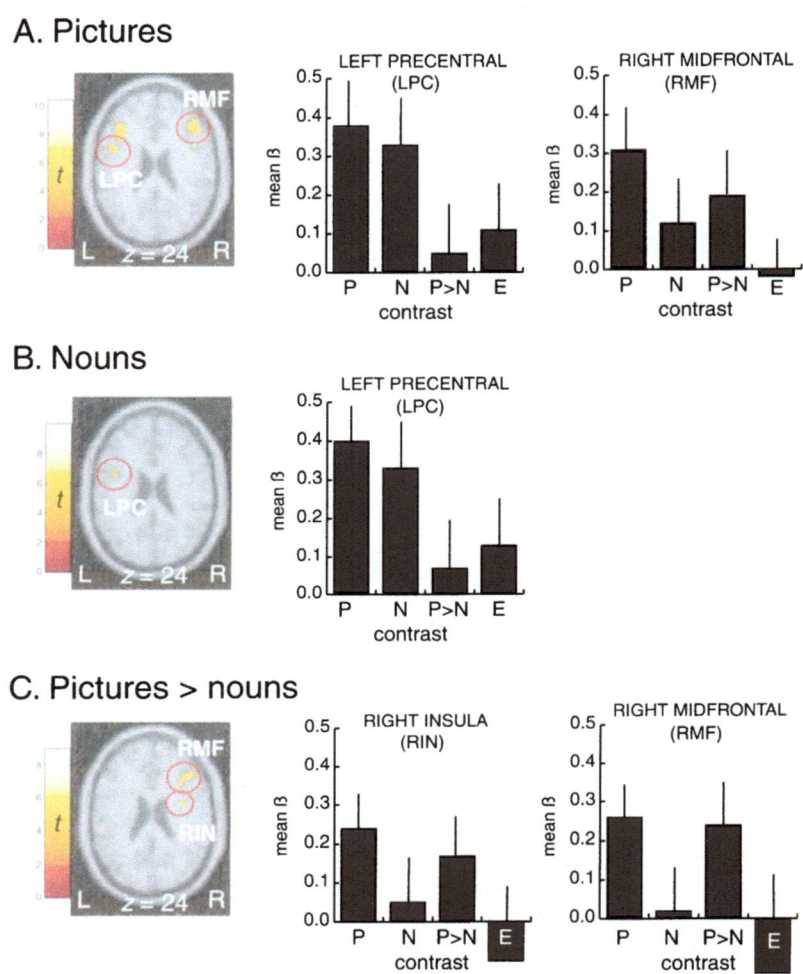

Figure 3. BOLD response in prefrontal cortex as a function of contrast. The data were thresholded at a value of $p < .0001$ (uncorrected), the minimum cluster size was 10 contiguous voxels, and the images shown are at $z = 24$. The graphs to the right of each image plot the mean ß value for the highlighted cluster across the four contrasts of interest: P = pictures imagery condition, N = nouns imagery condition, P > N = the direct comparison between the two imagery conditions, and E = visual encoding condition. These data suggest that the left precentral region (LPC) was significantly active in both the pictures (**A**) and nouns (**B**) conditions, but that the right midfrontal region (RMF) and right insula (RIN) were only active in the pictures condition (**C**). The statistical results are overlaid on the single-subject T1 anatomical image provided in SPM99. Error bars show 1 standard deviation.

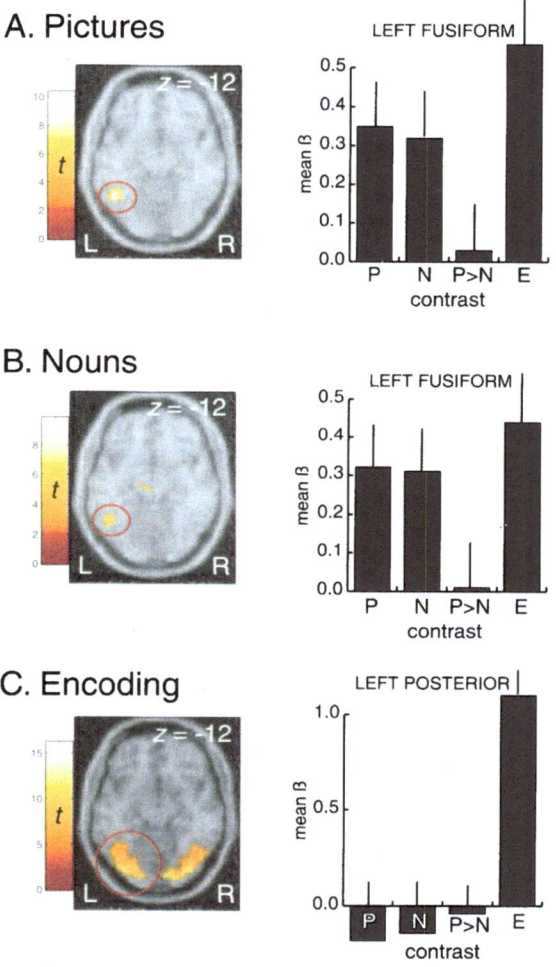

Figure 4. BOLD response in ventral temporal cortex as a function of contrast. The data were thresholded at a value of $p < .0001$ (uncorrected), the minimum cluster size was 10 contiguous voxels, and the images shown are at $z = -12$. The graphs to the right of each image plot the mean ß value for the highlighted cluster across the four contrasts of interest: P = pictures imagery condition, N = nouns imagery condition, P > N = the direct comparison between the two imagery conditions, and E = visual encoding condition. These data indicate that a common region of the left fusiform gyrus was significantly active in both the pictures **(A)** and nouns **(B)** conditions. The visual encoding condition produced much more widespread activation in visual cortex **(C)**. The statistical results are overlaid on the single-subject T1 anatomical image provided in SPM99. Error bars show 1 standard deviation.

encoding condition. Consistent with this interpretation, of the 42 voxels in the left fusiform gyrus activated during both imagery conditions, 23 of these voxels were also activated during the encoding condition. However, that imagery led to activation only in a small portion of visual cortex and is highlighted in Figure 4c, which shows both the anatomic extent of activation in visual cortex during visual stimulation, and the mean magnitude of response in visually activated cortex across all contrasts of interest.

Notably, there was no imagery-related activation in the region of MOC at the ROI criteria threshold of $p < .0001$ (uncorrected). Given the wide interest in understanding the behaviour of this region during imagery, we re-examined voxels in MOC at less conservative statistical thresholds. Even at a t probability value of $p < .01$ (uncorrected) there were no significant voxels in MOC in the pictures, nouns, or encoding contrasts. To better understand this null result in the group data, we then looked at the single-subject BOLD responses in this region

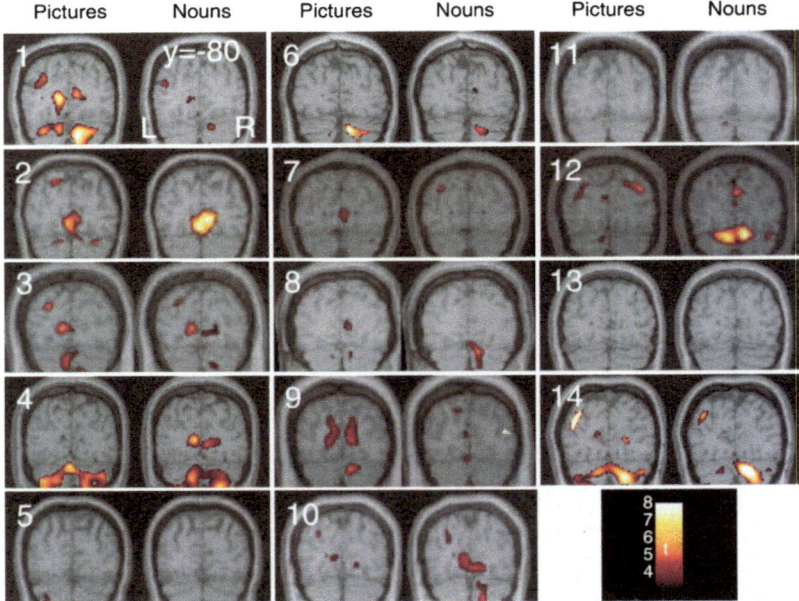

Figure 5.   Single-subject BOLD responses in MOC. The data were thresholded at a value of $p < .001$ (uncorrected), there was no minimum cluster size, and all images are shown at $y = -80$. For each subject, the BOLD response in this slice plane is shown as a function of contrast (pictures and nouns), with the individual participants identified via the number in the upper left-hand corner of each pair of images. These single-subject images reveal the wide individual variability in the BOLD response in MOC during the two imagery conditions. The data shown are spatially normalised and statistical overlaid on each subjects' normalised anatomical image. Cluster statistics are reported in Table 3.

by contrast (pictures and nouns). As shown in Figure 5, there was wide variance across participants in terms of whether there were significant voxel clusters in the MOC region in either one or both contrasts at a threshold of $p < .001$ (uncorrected). Talairach coordinates and statistics for these single-subject clusters are reported in Table 3. Importantly, not only does the variance across participants in the MOC BOLD response explain the lack of a significant effect in the group data, it is consistent with the growing belief that there is a high degree of individual variability in MOC activation during imagery.

TABLE 3
Significant voxel clusters in the medial occipital (MOC) region, by subject and contrast

Subject	P_task > P_rest					N_task > N_rest				
	x	y	z	k	t	x	y	z	k	t
1	−9	−75	6	4397	7 60	−9	−84	3	32	3.87
	12	−75	6	220	7.60					
2	6	−87	−3	461	6.80	6	−84	3	1137	6.60
3	−12	−84	3	226	5.41	−12	−81	3	219	4.90
						18	−81	−3		3.65
4			no clusters			0	−99	0	812	6.19
5			no clusters					no clusters		
6			no clusters			12	−78	12	107	3.90
7	6	−84	−3	198	4.49	6	−90	6	10	3.23*
8	9	−90	12	108	4.53	6	−90	12	13	3.77
9	−12	−81	9	1681	4.17	0	−96	0	121	4.89
	9	−84	6		5.17					
10	−12	−84	0	23	3.88	0	−84	−9	202	5.26
	18	−81	−6	23	3.68					
11			no clusters					no clusters		
12	−9	−78	6	18	3.04*	−12	−72	6	2039	4.60
	12	−81	12	1301	3.15*					
13			no clusters					no clusters		
14	−15	−78	12	30315	6.94			no clusters		
	21	−78	9		5.29					

Coordinates are in Talairach space, t values are for the local maxima in the MOC region within each cluster, and the minimum cluster size k was 10 voxels. Voxel clusters are reported at $p < .001$ (uncorrected), except those designated with an asterisk (*), which were clusters that were found to be significant only at a more permissive threshold ($p < .005$; uncorrected). If only one k value is reported for a pair of maxima, those maxima were in a contiguous voxel cluster at the reported threshold. P = pictures, N = nouns.

DISCUSSION

The data shown in Figure 3 suggest that the two imagery tasks invoked different retrieval processes in frontal cortex. While activations were comparable between conditions in the region of the left precentral gyrus, there were activations in both the right midfrontal and right insula regions during the pictures condition that were absent in the nouns condition. Importantly, this finding parallels a large corpus of evidence from the memory literature indicating that retrieval of temporally unique (or episodic) events engages processes in RFC that are typically not engaged during retrieval of more semantic-based information (e.g., Buckner et al., 1996; Cabeza et al., 1997; Düzel et al., 1999; Fletcher et al., 1995; Gabrieli et al., 1996; Haxby et al., 1996; Nyberg et al., 2000; Schacter et al., 1996; Tulving et al., 1994; Wagner et al., 1998). Although it remains an open question how to best characterise the functional nature of retrieval-related processing in RFC (e.g., Buckner & Wheeler, 2001; Koechlin, Basso, Pietrini, Panzer, & Grafman, 1999), the key point here is that processing in this region was differentially engaged in the two imagery conditions.[1]

Given the effect of imagery condition on retrieval processing, was there a corresponding difference between conditions in the pattern of visuocortical reactivation? The short answer is no. In both imagery conditions the same region of the left fusiform gyrus showed increased activation during imagery epochs relative to rest epochs (Figure 4). Indeed, there was substantial overlap in the two fusiform clusters, as quantified by the number of voxels showing above threshold activation in both conditions (see Results). That left ventral temporal cortex was engaged during imagery parallels the results of prior studies that have also shown activation in this region during imagery-related tasks (e.g., D'Esposito et al., 1997; Mellet et al., 1998b; Wheeler et al., 2000). The common fusiform response between conditions supports the argument that, despite the lack of an overt behavioural measure of task performance on each imagery attempt, both tasks did in fact lead to mental imagery. The data are thus relatively unambiguous in suggesting that despite apparent differences in the strategic retrieval mechanisms engaged during imagery generation, a common

---

[1] Given the lack of a direct behavioural measure of imagery performance in each condition, we cannot eliminate the possibility that there were common retrieval strategies used between conditions, at least for some items. However, the differential pattern of the bold response in frontal cortex indicates that, on average, there was in fact a difference in the retrieval strategies used between the two imagery conditions. Nevertheless, although we attribute these frontal differences between the pictures and nouns conditions to strategic processes associated with "episodic" and "semantic" retrieval, respectively, there may be additional contributing factors to consider as well. For example, the items imaged in the pictures condition may have been more like specific exemplars, while the items imaged in the nouns condition may have been more "prototypic" in nature. If so, there would be greater likelihood of individual variability in terms of imagery content generated in the nouns condition, in that there may be variance across participants in what passes as a prototypic image for a given object.

region of visual cortex was reactivated by the information retrieved from memory.

The data thus support the conclusion that a common visuocortical network was activated when the content of imagery was being held constant but the retrieval demands were varied. However, we stress that other factors are quite capable of influencing the pattern of cortical reactivation during imagery. For instance, imagery of spatial information is more likely to engage processing in parietal rather than ventral temporal cortex (e.g., Cohen et al., 1996; Mellet, Tzourio, Crivello, Joliot, Denis, & Mazoyer, 1996; Moscovitch, Kapur, Köhler, & Houle, 1995; see Mellet et al., 1998a). Likewise, visualising different categories of objects (e.g., faces vs. houses) has been shown to activate corresponding category-specific regions of ventral temporal cortex (e.g., Ishai et al., 2000; O'Craven & Kanwisher, 2000), and comparisons between visual and auditory imagery demonstrate that sensory-specific imagery content reactivates sensory-specific cortex (e.g., Wheeler et al., 2000). Common across these studies have been paradigms that vary the qualitative content of imagery between conditions in order to examine how it influences cortical reactivation.

In contrast, the experiment here demonstrates that if the content of imagery is held constant, reactivation of ventral temporal cortex appears to remain unaffected despite strategic changes in the memory retrieval processes used to generate that content. The finding closely parallels the results of Mellet et al. (2000), who showed that differences in encoding strategies also appear to have little influence on the network of posterior cortical regions activated during imagery. Our data are also consistent with the proposal that imagery content is perhaps the most decisive factor in determining the pattern of imagery-related activation in posterior cortex (e.g., Behrmann, 2000; Kosslyn & Thompson, 2000; Mellet et al., 1998a; Thompson & Kosslyn, 2000). As such, it remains an open question whether imagery-related activity in MOC may be labile to modulation by retrieval processes under conditions more suitable for observing task-related imagery effects in that region.

Although the focus of our study has been on determining the extent to which memory retrieval modulates visual cortical activity during imagery, the region of left fusiform gyrus found to be active in both imagery conditions is consistent with a wider network of posterior cortical areas that have been implicated in the interplay between memory and imagery (see Thompson & Kosslyn, 2000). In particular, both imagery tasks led to activation in the same pair of regions in left parietal cortex, namely the left inferior parietal lobule and left intraparietal sulcus (Figure 6). This finding is consistent with reports that left parietal regions are an integral component of the network of cortical areas involved in memory retrieval (e.g., Buckner & Wheeler, 2001; Habib & Lepage, 1999; Rugg & Wilding, 2000; see also Tomita, Ohbayashi, Nakahara, Hasegawa, & Miyashita, 1999) as well as visual imagery (e.g., Ishai et al., 2000; Mellet et al., 1998a). The common thread running through these discussions is that parietal regions are engaged during the retrieval attempt itself, and during the "top-down" reactivation of sensory cortex (if retrieval is successful).

Taken in this light, perhaps the least contentious conclusion to draw from the data in Figure 6 is that both the left inferior parietal lobule and left intraparietal sulcus were comparably involved in the two imagery tasks (see also Figure 2C). However, the data also provide partial evidence in support of the proposal of Mellet et al. (1998a) that this region is differentially more involved in imagery tied to episodic retrieval. The magnitude (ß) and anatomical extent of the response in the left intraparietal sulcus appeared to be larger in the pictures task relative to the nouns task (see Table 2). There was also evidence in the pictures > nouns contrast that the right inferior parietal lobule and precuneus were more active in the pictures condition as well. We offer these data as potential points of

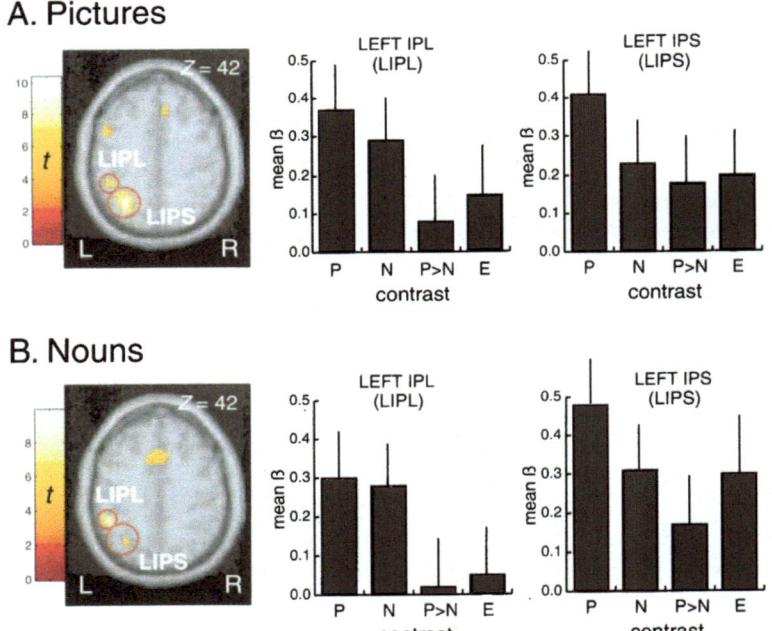

Figure 6. BOLD response in parietal cortex as a function of contrast. The data were thresholded at a value of $p < .0001$ (uncorrected), the minimum cluster size was 10 contiguous voxels, and all images shown are at $z = 42$. The graphs to the right of each image plot the mean ß value for the highlighted cluster across the four contrasts of interest: P = pictures imagery condition, N = nouns imagery condition, P > N = the direct comparison between the two imagery conditions, and E = visual encoding condition. These data suggest that common regions of the left inferior parietal lobule (LIPL) and the left intraparietal sulcus (LIPS) were significantly active in both the pictures **(A)** and nouns **(B)** conditions. The statistical results are overlaid on the single-subject T1 anatomical image provided in SPM99. Error bars show 1 standard deviation.

interest for future investigations focusing on the role of parietal cortex in memory retrieval and visual imagery.

At a more global level, one of the long-standing issues in the imagery literature has been whether there is cerebral hemisphere specialisation in the processes mediating visual imagery (e.g., Behrmann, 2000; Farah, 1995; Kosslyn, 1988; Kosslyn, Maljkovic, Hamilton, Horwitz, & Thompson, 1995a; Mellet et al., 1998a). The data in Figures 2C and 3C suggest that, in general, what was common between imagery conditions was processing in the left hemisphere and what was different between imagery conditions was processing in the right hemisphere. As such, our results are consistent with the proposition that a common network of areas in the left hemisphere were engaged during the two imagery conditions, including prefrontal, lateral parietal, and ventral temporal regions. If so, it raises the question of whether task manipulations that influence retrieval processing in left frontal cortex (e.g., repetition priming) would lead to corresponding changes in processing in the left hemisphere network implicated in the current study.

In conclusion, there are clear and important links between the neural systems we use to retrieve stored information and the systems we use to visualise an item that has been retrieved (e.g., Gonsalves & Paller, 2000; Ishai & Sagi, 1997; Mellet et al., 1998a; Wheeler et al., 2000). The data reported here speak directly to these links. From the memory perspective our results suggest that the segregation of strategic retrieval processes in frontal cortex does not extend to the visual areas activated during visual imagery. Rather, dissociable retrieval processes in frontal cortex appear to engage a common network of temporal and parietal areas when the intention of retrieval is to generate a visual mental image. In this sense, what the mind's eye sees during imagery appears to be unaffected by changes in the strategic processes in frontal cortex used to retrieve imagery content from memory.

PrEview proof published online May 2004

REFERENCES

Aguirre, G. K., Zarahn, E., & D'Esposito, M. (1998). The inferential impact of global signal covariates in functional neuroimaging analyses. *NeuroImage, 8*, 302–306.

Behrmann, M. (2000). The mind's eye mapped onto the brain's matter. *Current Directions in Psychological Science, 9*, 50–54.

Brewer, W. F., & Pani, J. R. (1996). Reports of mental imagery retrieval from long-term memory. *Consciousness and Cognition, 5*, 265–287.

Buckner, R. L., Raichle, M. E., Miezin, F. M., & Petersen, S. E. (1996). Functional anatomic studies of memory retrieval for auditory words and visual pictures. *Journal of Neuroscience, 16*, 6219–6235.

Buckner, R. L., & Wheeler, M. E. (2001). The cognitive neuroscience of remembering. *Nature Reviews Neuroscience, 2*, 624–634.

Cabeza, R., Kapur, S., Craik, F. I. M., McIntosh, A. R., Houle, S., & Tulving, E. (1997). Functional neuroanatomy of recall and recognition: A PET study of episodic memory. *Journal of Cognitive Neuroscience*, *9*, 254–265.

Cohen, M. S., Kosslyn, S. M., Breiter, H. C., DiGirolamo, G. J., Thompson, W. L., Anderson, A. K., Bookheimer, S. Y., Rosen, B. R., & Belliveau, J. W. (1996). Changes in cortical activity during mental rotation: A mapping study using functional magnetic resonance imaging. *Brain*, *119*, 89–100.

Denis, M., Goncalves, M. R., & Memmi, D. (1995). Mental scanning of visual images generated from verbal descriptions: Toward a model of image accuracy. *Neuropsychologia*, *33*, 1511–1530.

Desjardins, A. E., Kiehl, K. A., & Liddle, P. F. (2001). Removal of confounding effects of global signal in functional MRI analyses. *NeuroImage*, *13*, 751–758.

D'Esposito, M., Detre, J. A., Aguirre, G. K., Stallcup, M., Alsop, D. C., Tippet, L. J., Farah, M. J. (1997). A functional MRI study of mental image generation. *Neuropsychologia*, *35*, 725–730.

Düzel, E., Cabeza, R., Picton, T. W., Yonelinas, A. P., Scheich, H., Heinze, H. J., & Tulving, E. (1999). Task-related and item-related brain processes of memory retrieval. *Proceedings of the National Academy of Sciences, USA*, *96*, 1794–1799.

Farah, M. J. (1995). Current issues in the neuropsychology of image generation. *Neuropsychologia*, *33*, 1455–1471.

Fletcher, P. C., Frith, C. D., Grasby, P. M., Shallice, T., Frackowiak, R. S. J., & Dolan, R. J. (1995). Brain systems for encoding and retrieval of auditory–verbal memory. *Brain*, *118*, 401–416.

Friston, K. J., Ashburner, J., Frith, C. D., Poline, J.-P., Heather, J. D., & Frackowiak, R. S. J. (1995a). Spatial registration and normalization of images. *Human Brain Mapping*, *2*, 165–189.

Friston, K. J., Holmes, A. P., Worsley, K. J., Poline, J.-P., Frith, C. D., & Frackowiak, R. S. J. (1995b). Statistical parametric maps in functional imaging: A general linear approach. *Human Brain Mapping*, *2*, 189–210.

Friston, K. J., Williams, S., Howard, R., Frackowiak, R. S., & Turner, R. (1996). Movement-related effects in fMRI time-series. *Magnetic Resonance in Medicine*, *35*, 346–355.

Gabrieli, J. D. E., Desmond, J. E., Demb, J. B., Wagner, A. D., Stone, M. V., Vaidya, C. J., & Glover, G. H. (1996). Functional magnetic resonance imaging of semantic memory processes in the frontal lobes. *Psychological Science*, *7*, 278–283.

Gonsalves, B., & Paller, K. A. (2000). Neural events that underlie remembering something that never happened. *Nature Neuroscience*, *3*, 1316–1321.

Habib, R., & Lepage, M. (1999). Novelty assessment in the brain. In E. Tulving (Ed.), *Memory, consciousness, and the brain*. Philadelphia: Psychology Press.

Haxby, J. V., Ungerleider, L. G., Horwitz, B., Maisog, J. M., Rapoport, S. I., & Grady, C. L. (1996). Face encoding and recognition in the human brain. *Proceedings of the National Academy of Sciences, USA*, *93*, 922–927.

Ishai, A., & Sagi, D. (1997). Visual imagery: Effects of short- and long-term memory. *Journal of Cognitive Neuroscience*, *9*, 734–742.

Ishai, A., Ungerleider, L. G., & Haxby, J. V. (2000). Distributed neural systems for the generation of visual images. *Neuron*, *28*, 979–990.

Kelley, W. M., Buckner, R. L., & Petersen, S. E. (1998). Response from Kelley, Buckner, & Petersen. *Trends in Cognitive Science*, *2*, 421.

Koechlin, E., Basso, G., Pietrini, P., Panzer, S., & Grafman, J. (1999). The role of the anterior prefrontal cortex in human cognition. *Nature*, *399*, 148–151.

Kosslyn, S. M. (1988). Aspects of a cognitive neuroscience of mental imagery. *Science*, *240*, 1621–1626.

Kosslyn, S. M., Alpert, N. M., Thompson, W. L., Maljkovic, V., Weise, S. B., Chabris, C. F., Hamilton, S. E., Rauch, S. L., & Buonanno, F. S. (1993). Visual mental imagery activates topographically organized visual cortex: PET investigations. *Journal of Cognitive Neuroscience*, *5*, 263–287.

Kosslyn, S. M., Ganis, G., & Thompson, W. L. (2001). Neural foundations of imagery. *Nature Reviews Neuroscience*, *2*, 635–642.

Kosslyn, S. M., Maljkovic, V., Hamilton, S. E., Horwitz, G., & Thompson, W. L. (1995a). Two types of image generation: Evidence for left and right hemisphere processes. *Neuropsychologia, 33,* 1485–1510.

Kosslyn, S. M., Pascual-Leone, A., Felician, O., Camposano, S., Keenan, J. P., Thompson, W. L., Ganis, G., Sukel, K. E., & Alpert, N. M. (1999). The role of area 17 in visual imagery: Convergent evidence from PET and rTMS. *Science, 284,* 167–170.

Kosslyn, S. M., & Thompson, W. L. (2000). Shared mechanisms in visual imagery and visual perception: Insights from cognitive neuroscience. In M. S. Gazzaniga (Ed.), *The new cognitive neurosciences* (2nd ed.). Cambridge, MA: MIT Press.

Kosslyn, S. M., Thompson, W. L., & Alpert, N. M. (1997). Neural systems shared by visual imagery and visual perception: A positron emission tomography study. *NeuroImage, 6,* 320–334.

Kosslyn, S. M., Thompson, W. L., Kim, I. J., & Alpert, N. M. (1995b). Topographical representations of mental images in primary visual cortex. *Nature, 378,* 496–498.

Krelman, G., Koch, C., & Fried, I. (2000). Imagery neurons in the human brain. *Nature, 408,* 357–361.

Le Bihan, D., Turner, R., Zeffiro, T. A., Cuénod, C. A., Jezzard, P., & Bonnerot, V. (1993). Activation of human primary visual cortex during visual recall: A magnetic resonance imaging study. *Proceedings of the National Academy of Sciences, USA, 90,* 11802–11805.

Mellet, E., Petit, L., Mazoyer, B., Denis, M., & Tzourio, N. (1998a). Reopening the mental imagery debate: Lessons from functional anatomy. *NeuroImage, 8,* 129–139.

Mellet, E., Tzourio, N., Crivello, F., Joliot, M., Denis, M., & Mazoyer, B. (1996). Functional anatomy of spatial mental imagery generated from verbal instructions. *Journal of Neuroscience, 16,* 6504–6512.

Mellet, E., Tzourio, N., Denis, M., & Mazoyer, B. (1998b). Cortical anatomy of mental imagery of concrete nouns based on their dictionary definition. *Neuroreport, 9,* 803–808.

Mellet, E., Tzourio-Mazoyer, N., Bricogne, S., Mazoyer, B., Kosslyn, S. M., & Denis, M. (2000). Functional anatomy of high-resolution visual mental imagery. *Journal of Cognitive Neuroscience, 12,* 98–109.

Moscovitch, M., Kapur, S., Köhler, S., & Houle, S. (1995). Distinct neural correlates of visual long-term memory for spatial location and object identity: A positron emission tomography study in humans. *Proceedings of the National Academy of Sciences, USA, 92,* 3721–3725.

Nyberg, L., Cabeza, R., & Tulving, E. (1998). Asymmetric frontal activation during episodic memory: What kind of specificity? *Trends in Cognitive Science, 2,* 419–420.

Nyberg, L., Habib, R., McIntosh, A. R., & Tulving, E. (2000). Reactivation of encoding-related brain activity during memory retrieval. *Proceedings of the National Academy of Sciences, USA, 97,* 11120–11124.

O'Craven, K. M., & Kanwisher, N. (2000). Mental imagery of faces and places activates corresponding stimulus-specific brain regions. *Journal of Cognitive Neuroscience, 12,* 1013–1023.

Roland, P. E., & Gulyás, B. (1994). Visual imagery and visual representation. *Trends in Neuroscience, 17,* 281–289.

Rugg, M. D., & Wilding, E. L. (2000). Retrieval processing and episodic memory. *Trends in Cognitive Science, 4,* 108–115.

Sakai, K., & Miyashita, Y. (1993). Memory and imagery in the temporal lobe. *Current Opinion in Neurobiology, 3,* 166–170.

Schacter, D. L., Alpert, N. M., Savage, C. R., Rauch, S. L., & Albert, M. S. (1996). Conscious recollection and the human hippocampal formation: Evidence from positron emission tomography. *Proceedings of the National Academy of Sciences, USA, 93,* 321–325.

Talairach, J., & Tournoux, P. (1988). *Co-planar stereotaxic atlas of the human brain.* New York: Thieme Medical Publishers.

Thompson, W. L., & Kosslyn, S. M. (2000). Neural systems activated during visual mental imagery: A review and meta-analyses. In W. Toga & J. C. Mazziotta (Eds.), *Brain mapping: The systems.* San Diego: Academic Press.

Thompson, W. L., Kosslyn, S. M., Sukel, K. E., & Alpert, N. M. (2001). Mental imagery of high- and low-resolution gratings activates area 17. *NeuroImage, 14,* 454–464.

Tomita, H., Ohbayashi, M., Nakahara, K., Hasegawa, I., & Miyashita, Y. (1999). Top-down signal from prefrontal cortex in executive control of memory retrieval. *Nature, 401,* 699–703.

Tulving, E., Kapur, S., Craik, F. I. M., Moscovitch, M., & Houle, S. (1994). Hemispheric encoding/ retrieval asymmetry in episodic memory: Positron emission tomography findings. *Proceedings of the National Academy of Sciences, USA, 91,* 2016–2020.

Wagner, A. D., Poldrack, R. A., Eldridge, L. L., Desmond, J. E., Glover, G. H., & Gabrieli, J. D. E. (1998). Material-specific lateralization of prefrontal activation during episodic encoding and retrieval. *Neuroreport, 9,* 3711–3717.

Wheeler, M. E., Petersen, S. E., & Buckner, R. L. (2000). Memory's echo: Vivid remembering reactivates sensory-specific cortex. *Proceedings of the National Academy of Sciences, USA, 97,* 11125–11129.

EUROPEAN JOURNAL OF COGNITIVE PSYCHOLOGY, 2004, *16* (5), 653–672

What clocks tell us about the neural correlates of spatial imagery

Luigi Trojano

Department of Psychology, Second University of Naples, Caserta, and Salvatore Maugeri Foundation, IRCCS, Institute of Telese, Italy

David E. J. Linden

Max-Planck-Institut für Hirnforschung, and Department of Psychiatry, Laboratory for Neurophysiology and Neuroimaging, Johann Wolfgang Goethe-Universität, Frankfurt, Germany, and School of Psychology, University of Wales, Bangor, UK

Elia Formisano and Rainer Goebel

Department of Cognitive Neuroscience, Faculty of Psychology, Maastricht University, The Netherlands

Alexander T. Sack

Department of Psychiatry, Laboratory for Neurophysiology and Neuroimaging, Johann Wolfgang Goethe-Universität, Frankfurt, Germany

Francesco Di Salle

Department of Neurological Sciences, Division of Neuroradiology, Federico II University, Naples, Italy

We review a series of experimental studies aimed at answering some critical questions about the neural basis of spatial imagery. Our group used functional magnetic resonance imaging (fMRI) to explore the neural correlates of an online behaviourally controlled spatial imagery task without need for visual presentation—the mental clock task. Subjects are asked to imagine pairs of times that are presented acoustically and to judge at which of the two times the clock hands form the greater angle. The cortical activation elicited by this task was contrasted with that obtained during other visual, perceptual, verbal, and spatial imagery tasks in several block design studies. Moreover, our group performed an event-related fMRI study on the clock task to investigate the representation of component cognitive processes in spatial imagery. The bulk of our findings demonstrates that

Correspondence should be addressed to Luigi Trojano, Department of Psychology, Second University of Naples, Via Vivaldi 43, 81100 Caserta, Italy. Email: luigi.trojano@unina2.it

© 2004 Psychology Press Ltd
http://www.tandf.co.uk/journals/pp/09541446.html   DOI: 10.1080/09541440340000510

cortical areas in the posterior parietal cortex (PPC), along the intraparietal sulcus, are robustly involved in spatial mental imagery and in other tasks requiring spatial transformations. PPC is bilaterally involved in different kinds of spatial judgement. Yet the degree to which right and left PPC are activated in different tasks is a function of task requirements. From event-related fMRI data we obtained evidence that left and right PPC are activated asynchronously during the clock task and this could reflect their different functional role in subserving cognitive components of visuospatial imagery.

A BRIEF OVERVIEW OF THE NEUROPSYCHOLOGY OF SPATIAL MENTAL IMAGERY

Many tasks have been used to study the ability to visualise objects in the mind. Some of them require subjects to represent mentally visual features of objects, while others explicitly require the processing of spatially coded information. In the neuropsychological literature, several brain-lesioned patients have been reported with selective deficits in the performance of visual or spatial imagery tasks. Levine, Warach, and Farah (1985) and Farah, Hammond, Levine, and Calvanio (1988) described a patient who had a specific impairment in performing visual imagery tasks concerning the colour, size, and shape of objects. This patient was, for example, unable to tell whether certain animals have long or short tails or to compare the outlines of the borders of the American states. Yet he could perform spatial imagery tasks like mental rotation of letters or 3-D abstract figures and knew perfectly the location of the states. Levine et al. (1985) had already reported a patient with the complementary imagery deficit, but an extensive description of a patient affected by a selective impairment of spatial imagery was offered by Luzzatti, Vecchi, Agazzi, Cesa-Bianchi, and Vergani (1998). This patient could draw from memory or describe objects and animals correctly, and answer questions about visual features of objects, but was unable to describe spatial relationships among elements of complex objects or among streets and squares of her hometown. Similarly, she failed in spatial imagery tasks that required the construction of imagined matrices or spatial configurations.

This neuropsychological evidence for a double dissociation between visual and spatial imagery tasks suggests that distinct cognitive processes are involved in the two kinds of imagery. This distinction parallels that established in the visual perception domain into an occipitotemporal (ventral) pathway responsible for object identification and an occipital-parietal (dorsal) pathway responsible for spatial processing (Ungerleider & Mishkin, 1982). Nonetheless, neuroanatomical findings in these patients did not provide stringent clues for the neural basis of spatial mental imagery. In fact, the patient with a selective impairment in visual imagery tasks described by Farah et al. (1988) had widespread bilateral temporo-occipital and right inferofrontal lesions, whereas the patients with selective impairment in spatial imagery tasks had bilateral parieto-occipital lesions (Levine et al., 1985) or a cortical atrophy that was more prominent in the right temporal lobe (Luzzatti et al., 1998).

FUNCTIONAL NEUROIMAGING STUDIES OF SPATIAL MENTAL IMAGERY

The issue of the neural basis of spatial imagery has been tackled by means of modern neuroimaging techniques in different experimental paradigms. In their recent empirical review of neuroimaging studies, Cabeza and Nyberg (2000) list several papers on spatial imagery, most of which employed visual presentations of stimuli that had to be mentally rotated to comply with task requirements (Alivisatos & Petrides, 1997; Cohen et al., 1996; Kosslyn, DiGirolamo, Thompson, & Alpert, 1998). Only a few studies investigated the entire process of spatial image generation and processing in the absence of visual stimulation. In the first (Mellet et al., 1995), subjects mentally explored a map memorised in previous learning sessions. In a second study (Mellet, Tzourio, Denis, & Mazoyer, 1996), subjects mentally assembled objects from spatial instructions they had heard. A third study required subjects to perform a mental navigation along routes previously memorised through a walk in the real environment (Ghaem et al., 1997).

In their recent critical meta-analysis of functional studies on imagery, Thompson and Kosslyn (2000) concluded that the activation patterns during imagery tasks depend strongly on the kind of task used, the type of the experimental paradigm, and the neuroimaging method. When the task requires spatial operations or when mental images have to be transformed, posterior parietal regions are likely to be activated, while primary visual cortex activation would be expected when tasks require detailed, high-resolution mental images. For instance, activation of posterior parietal cortex (PPC) has been observed in conjunction with the spatial transformation of visually presented stimuli (Alivisatos & Petrides, 1997; Cohen et al., 1996). In a recent PET study of mental rotation (Alivisatos & Petrides, 1997), right PPC was seen to participate in the processing of mirror images of letters or digits. Activation of the superior parietal lobule in both hemispheres has been described in an fMRI study of the analysis of spatially transformed words and phrases, which also distinguished this spatial transformation-related activation from general attentional effects (Goebel, Linden, Lanfermann, Zanella, & Singer, 1998b). The construction of three-dimensional mental images from auditory instructions, as studied by PET (Mellet, Tzourio, Crivello, Joliot, Denis, & Mazoyer, 1996), involved a distributed system of frontal, occipital, and parietal areas. The parietal activation, however, was most prominent in the right precuneus and supramarginal gyrus and did not involve the PPC.

The majority of earlier studies could not monitor subjects' performances online during the execution of the task, and some involved visual presentation of stimuli, generating the possible confound of saccade-related activation in the parietal lobe (Milner & Goodale, 1995). Our group used fMRI to explore the neural correlates of an online behaviourally controlled spatial imagery task without need for visual presentation. In some subjects we also controlled eye movements during the scanning session. The experimental task was derived from the mental clock task (Grossi, Angelini, Pecchinenda, & Pizzamiglio, 1993; Grossi, Modafferi, Pelosi, & Trojano, 1989; Paivio, 1978). Subjects are asked to imagine pairs of times that are presented acoustically and to judge at which of the two times the clock hands form the greater angle. Paivio (1978) demonstrated that when subjects have to judge the difference between the angles formed by the hour and the minute hand on an imagined clock face, they report using imagery and show a symbolic distance effect: reaction time increases as angular size difference decreases. The clock task is particularly suitable for the functional magnetic resonance imaging (fMRI) investigation of mental imagery because it involves a behavioural control that can be performed online during scanning and has the specific advantage that pairs of digital clock times can be presented visually to compare performance and cerebral activation between an imagery and a closely matched visual perceptual condition. Moreover, the task permits the assessment of imagery abilities separately for each visual hemifield. The clock task has already been used in neuropsychological studies on brain-lesioned patients with selective imagery defects or with neglect-related spatial deficits (Grossi et al., 1989, 1993).

We planned a series of experimental studies aimed to clarify the pattern of cortical activation during the execution of the mental clock task. In particular, we aimed at answering a series of critical questions about the neural basis of spatial imagery.

WHICH CORTICAL NETWORK IS INVOLVED IN SPATIAL IMAGERY AND IS IT SHARED WITH VISUAL PERCEPTION?

In the first study (Trojano et al., 2000) the mental clock task was used in two experiments that addressed the cortical network involved in spatial imagery and its relationship to perceptual visuospatial processing. The two experiments provided converging evidence for the involvement of the PPC of both cerebral hemispheres in spatial imagery. Four healthy subjects participated in the second experiment, where we compared the activity during the mental clock task (*imagery*) to the same operation performed on visually presented clocks (*perception*) and to a nonspatial control task (*syllable counting*), whose attentional load proved comparable to that of the *imagery* task. The MR scanner used for imaging was a 1.5 T whole body superconducting system (MAGNETOM Vision, Siemens Medical Systems, Erlangen, Germany) equipped with a standard head coil, an active shielded gradient coil (25 mT/m) and Echo Planar (EPI) sequences for ultrafast MR imaging. For functional imaging, we used a BOLD (blood oxygenation level-dependent) sensitive single shot EPI sequence (echo time, TE = 66 ms; flip angle, FA = 90°; matrix size = 128 × 128, voxel dimensions = 1.4 mm × 1.4 mm × 4 mm) with an interscan temporal spacing of 5 s. Stimuli were presented in a block design.

In the mental clock task, subjects had to imagine pairs of analogue clock faces based on the times that were presented verbally by the examiner (e.g., 9.30 and 10.00; ISI = 1 s), and to judge at which of the two times the clock hands form the greater angle (imagery condition). In half stimuli, hours had to be imagined on the right half of the clock face (e.g., 3.00), and in the remaining half hours occupied the left half of the dial (e.g., 9.00); presentation order was randomised. During the syllable counting condition, we asked subjects to count the syllables of each pair of times and to report whether the total syllable number was odd or even. In the perception condition we used pairs of analogue clock faces; the clock faces of each pair were generated on a computer screen and projected one at a time (ISI = 1 s) in the central visual field.

In all the experimental conditions, half of the subjects had to push a button with their right index finger to choose the first stimulus of each pair as the correct response, or their left index finger to choose the second stimulus; in the remaining subjects, response modality was reversed. Subjects' responses were registered by an optic fibre answer box and analysed for speed and accuracy. During the imagery and perception condition, material and response modality were the same. In the latter case, however, the pairs of times were presented visually to the subject while in the imagery condition they had to be visualised mentally. In the syllable counting condition, material, presentation and response modality were the same as in the imagery task, but here a verbal–phonological judgement was required. Subjects were asked to keep their eyes open during the scanning session and foveate a fixation cross in order to avoid eye movements.

Data analysis, registration, and surface-based visualisation were performed with the fMRI software package BrainVoyager (Goebel & Singer, 1999). The statistical analysis of the BOLD signal (for review see Di Salle et al., 1999) time courses was based on the general linear model of the experiment. In this approach, each experimental condition (i.e., imagery, perception, syllable counting) is considered an effect of interest. The corresponding time points, convolved with a haemodynamic response function modelling the characteristics of the BOLD response, constitute the predictors of the model. The visualisation tools of the BrainVoyager software permit the reconstruction of the cortical surface of the subject's brain on the basis of a high-resolution 3-D anatomical MR data set. Colour-coded statistical maps ($p' < 10-3$ corrected) can then be visualised conventionally on individual slices through the brain or on surface representations. The display of functional maps on inflated or flattened hemispheres allows the topographic representation of the three-dimensional pattern of cortical activation without loss of the lobular structure of the telencephalon

(Goebel, Khorram-Sefat, Muckli, Hacker, & Singer, 1998a; Linden, 2002; Linden et al., 1999).

Behavioural results showed that the imagery (mean correct response time: 2517 ± 860 ms; 45.5 ± 6.4 correct responses out of 48 trials) and syllable counting conditions (mean correct response time: 2940 ± 1039 ms; 39.5 ± 4.9 correct responses) had equivalent processing load (no significant differences on Mann-Whitney test), while the perception condition proved to be significantly simpler than the others, both for response accuracy (47.1 ± 0.8 correct responses) and reaction times (mean correct response time: 1433 ± 618 ms). Multiple regression analysis of the BOLD time course revealed a significantly higher activation of the intraparietal sulcus (IPS) region of the posterior parietal cortex (PPC) for the execution of the mental clock task compared to the syllable counting condition (Figure 1A). The comparison between the perception and baseline conditions showed an activation of posterior parietal cortex very similar to that observed during the imagery condition. However, in the contrast between the imagery and perception conditions (Figure 1B) no activation was evident in PPC. In the imagery condition increased activity was present in right prefrontal cortex and in mesial frontal areas bilaterally, while occipital and inferior temporal areas were activated bilaterally in the perception condition (see also Table 1).

The most striking result of this study is that cortical activation (as measured by an increase of the fMRI BOLD signal) during the mental clock task was most prominent in the posterior parietal lobes of both hemispheres. This activation can be regarded as specific for the visuospatial operations because it was observed in both visuospatial tasks (in the imagery and perceptual domain), but not in a nonvisuospatial control task that involved the same acoustically presented material and was of equivalent difficulty as the imagery task. The direct contrast between the perception and imagery conditions (i.e., the clock task performed on visually presented and mentally imagined material, respectively) yielded no significant activation differences in the PPC. This indicates that this area is recruited to a comparable extent for visuospatial imagery and perceptual processing.

Interestingly, no similar overlap of activation was observed in occipito-temporal cortex. The perception condition (spatial matching of visually presented clocks), compared to the fixation baseline, yielded very prominent bilateral activation of the inferior temporal and the inferior and lateral occipital lobes. This occipitotemporal activation was still observed when the perception condition was contrasted with the imagery condition. These areas, which include the area LO and the fusiform gyri, have been shown to be involved in the processing of visual objects (Malach et al., 1995). They are assumed to form part of the ventral pathway of visual processing (Ungerleider & Mishkin, 1982), while the posterior parietal cortex has been assigned a role in the dorsal pathway responsible for the processing of visual motion and space (Goebel et al., 1998b; Ungerleider & Haxby, 1994).

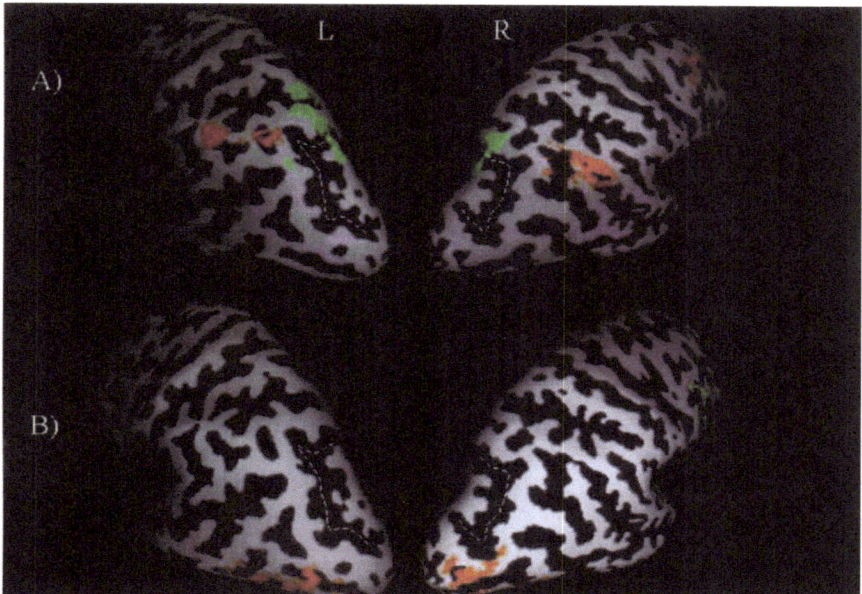

Figure 1. Statistical results of the first block design study of the mental clock task (Trojano et al., 2000) were visualised through projecting 3-D statistical maps on inflated surface reconstructions of the cortical sheet (posterior view, the dotted lines indicate the IPS). For significantly activated voxels, the relative contribution RC between two selected sets of conditions in explaining the variance of a voxel time course were computed as $RC = (b1 - b2)/(b1 + b2)$ where bi is the sum of the estimates of the standardised regression coefficients of all conditions included in set 1. The RC index was visualised with a red–green pseudocolour scale. An RC value of 1 (red) indicates that a voxel time course is solely explained with predictor set 1, whereas an RC value of -1 (green) indicates that a voxel time course is explained solely with predictor set 2. A RC value of 0 indicates that a voxel time course is explained with an equal contribution of both predictor sets. In the relative contribution maps, only RC values greater than 0.7 were visualised. **(A)** The relative contribution of the imagery (green) and syllable counting (red) predictors to the explanation of the variance of the cortical BOLD signal change. Note that imagery-related activation is apparent along the IPS bilaterally while syllable counting involved the inferior parietal cortex (IPL) bilaterally and the right DLPFC. **(B)** An analogous relative contribution map for the imagery (green) and perception (red) predictors. Note that no imagery-related activation was observed in occipitotemporal areas.

The white dotted line corresponds to the intraparietal sulcus and its main branches. Reprinted with permission of Oxford University Press (Trojano et al., 2000).

Inferior temporal areas were also found to be involved in visual mental imagery, particularly when object properties had to be encoded as in the case of imagery of faces and places (O'Craven & Kanwisher, 2000). In our study of spatial imagery, however, the ventral pathway was recruited exclusively during the perceptual condition and convergence of the cortical processing streams for visuospatial processing in perception and imagery was only observed at the level

TABLE 1

Location and extension of contrasts between the imagery and the control conditions (data from Trojano et al., 2000)

Anatomical area	BA	Imagery (I) vs. Syllables (S)					Imagery (I) vs. Perception (P)				
		Task	x	y	z	Size	Task	x	y	z	Size
Left posterior parietal cortex	7	I	−19	−67	48	1010	—				
Right posterior parietal cortex	7	I	17	−64	43	726	—				
Left perisylvian cortex	45/ins	S	−49	15	0	507	—				
Right perisylvian cortex	45/ins	S	44	13	1	984	—				
Left inferior parietal lobule	39/40	S	−45	−46	44	612	—				
Right inferior parietal lobule	39/40	S	52	−45	43	532	—				
Left superior frontal gyrus	6/8	—					I	−3	28	37	171
Right superior frontal gyrus	6/8	—					I	4	28	40	625
Right prefrontal cortex	9	S	43	21	39	662	I	53	13	26	435
Left occipitotemporal cortex	37/19	—					P	−45	−57	−9	556
Right occipitotemporal cortex	37/19	—					P	44	−65	−12	1181
Left middle occipital gyrus	19	—					P	−35	−79	3	515
Right middle occipital gyrus	19	—					P	32	−80	2	401

The position of each area is given as the Talairach coordinates of the centre of mass of the supra-threshold ($p' < 10^{-3}$, corrected) clusters of the multisubject analysis. Size = number of voxels ($1 \times 1 \times 1$ mm) of each area.

of the dorsal pathway. This dissociation lends further support to the view that the degree of recruitment of the cortical visual subsystems for mental imagery very much depends on the characteristics of the task, particularly the requirements on detailed image inspection, spatial transformation, and encoding of object properties (Thompson & Kosslyn, 2000).

The results of our study of the mental clock task indicate that while there is convergence of the cortical processing streams for visuospatial processing in perception and imagery at the level of the dorsal pathway, the ventral pathway is recruited exclusively during the perceptual condition. The area in the superior PPC is active when the spatial task is performed on mental images, even in the absence of any visual stimulation. This similarity of activation patterns can be explained in two ways. First, the superior IPS might be instrumental in the .computation of spatial transformations, regardless of whether the material is present in the visual field or merely as a mental image. Alternatively, any spatial transformation task, whether it involves visually perceived or imagined material, or indeed tactile stimulation (Sathian, Zangaladze, Hoffmann, & Grafton, 1997) might require the implicit generation of mental visual representations (Kosslyn & Sussmann, 1995).

DO DIFFERENT KINDS OF SPATIAL IMAGERY TASKS RELY ON DIFFERENT CORTICAL NETWORKS?

Our high-resolution fMRI findings demonstrated that posterior parietal cortex is strongly involved in the processing of spatially coded material in the imagery domain. The comparison of our results with those of recent studies of spatial transformations of visually presented material indicates that the analysis of visual space in perception and imagery has a common neural basis in the parietal lobes. It can be suggested that the neural networks involved in the processes of spatial processing are shared by several cognitive functions, including visuo-spatial imagery. In a subsequent study we aimed to clarify whether different parts of the PPC are involved in different kinds of spatial imagery tasks.

Current theoretical models predict that two different kinds of spatial encoding proceed in parallel. One process encodes discrete (''categorical'') spatial relations, those easily described by verbal locatives like left/right or above/below, while the other encodes metric (''coordinate'') spatial relations, representing precise, quantitative aspects of the spatial relationships (Kosslyn, 1994). Both cerebral hemispheres participate in spatial processing of visual input, but each seems to be specialised for a particular kind of spatial processing. The left hemisphere would be relatively faster than the right at encoding ''categorical'' spatial relations, while the right hemisphere would be superior at encoding metric (''coordinate'') spatial relations (Brown & Kosslyn, 1993; Kosslyn, 1987). It has been suggested that the categorical/coordinate dichotomy may apply also to the visual imagery domain (Kosslyn, Maljkovic, Hamilton, Horwitz, & Thompson, 1995; Michimata, 1997).

The mental clock task as described above represents a paradigm for "coordinate" judgements in the imagery domain because it requires the generation of multipart mental images and a subsequent spatial metric comparison task (Michimata, 1997; Trojano & Grossi, 1994). In a block-design experiment we contrasted the "coordinate" clock task with a "categorical" task applied to the same clock stimuli (Trojano et al., 2002). For the "categorical" task we asked subjects to imagine analogue clock faces according to the procedure of the classical mental clock task. However, this time they had to judge whether both hands lay in a given half (upper, lower, right, or left) of the clock face. Both tasks share several cognitive processes: auditory processing of verbal instructions, image generation, image maintenance and scanning, and response selection procedures. The comparison between the two tasks, and that between each task and a third experimental condition employing the same auditorily presented verbal material and a comparable working memory load, should reveal whether the posterior parietal cortex is involved in both kinds of spatial processing and, moreover, whether any lateralisation of cortical activation corresponds to the categorical/coordinate dichotomy in the imagery domain (Michimata, 1997).

Seven healthy right-handed postgraduate students participated in the study. The experimental paradigm included the clock task given as in the previous study (*coordinate* condition). In the *categorical* condition, subjects were asked to imagine an analogue clock face showing the time verbally presented by the examiner. After each verbal presentation of a time, subjects heard a cue indicating one half of the clock face (left, right, upper, or lower; ISI = 1 s) and they had to judge whether both hands lay in the cued half of the clock face (congruent trials) or not (noncongruent trials). For noncongruent trials, times were chosen that would correspond to a different cue. This choice was made to discourage subjects from resorting to verbal labels, and compel them to form mental images in response to all clock stimuli. We also included a nonspatial *control* condition, in which we asked subjects to count the syllables of each of the auditorily presented pairs of times and to report whether the total syllable number was odd or even. The three conditions were alternated in blocks of eight trials, and the categorical and the coordinate conditions were alternated in the sequence of stimulation conditions, with the control task always following the two imagery tasks. Subjects' responses were registered by an optic-fibre answer box and analysed for accuracy and response times. Subjects were asked to keep their eyes open during the scanning session and foveate a fixation cross in order to avoid eye movements.

MR hardware and sequences were the same as in the previous study. Data analysis, registration, and surface-based visualisation were performed with the fMRI software package BrainVoyager (Goebel & Singer, 1999). The statistical analysis of the BOLD time courses, limited to cortical voxels, was based on the general linear model of the experiment with the *categorical* and the *coordinate* imagery tasks, and the nonspatial *control* condition (syllable counting) as the effects of interest. The global level of the signal time courses in each session was considered to be a confounding effect. Statistical results ($p' < 10^{-3}$ corrected) were then visualised through projecting 3-D statistical maps on surface reconstruction of the cortical sheet.

Analysis of behavioural data showed that the syllable counting task proved to be the most difficult task (mean correct reaction time: 2788 ± 635 ms; $76.2 \pm 12.7\%$ of correct responses), while the categorical (mean correct reaction time: 2450 ± 396 ms; $84.8 \pm 3.9\%$ of correct responses) and the coordinate (mean correct reaction time: 2413 ± 416 ms; $83.2 \pm 6.7\%$ of correct responses) spatial judgement tasks yielded similar results. The three experimental conditions did not differ significantly in their behavioural measures (Kruskal-Wallis test). As for fMRI data, the contrasts between the *categorical* and the *coordinate* conditions and the *control* task yielded similar, but not overlapping, cortical activation patterns (Table 2).

Both spatial imagery tasks activated the superior parietal lobule bilaterally. Moreover, activated cortical areas were also seen along the anterior part of the intraparietal sulcus, extending into the inferior parietal lobule bilaterally in the *coordinate* task, and only on the left side in the *categorical* task. The relative contribution maps of the spatial imagery tasks (Figure 2) suggested that the categorical and the coordinate processing of spatial mental images shared a common region of activation in the superior parietal lobule, but with some differences between each other. The areas in the superior parietal lobule showed a relatively lateralised pattern of activation, with a higher (but not exclusive) contribution of the right side during the *coordinate* task, and a higher contribution of the left during the *categorical* task. Both tasks activated the angular gyrus bilaterally, in the depth of the anterior part of intraparietal sulcus; the

TABLE 2

Location and extension of contrasts between the coordinate and the categorical spatial imagery task (data from Trojano et al., 2002)

	BA	Side	*Coordinate judgement*				*Categorical judgement*			
			x	*y*	*z*	*Size*	*x*	*y*	*z*	*Size*
Superior parietal lobule	7	L	−17	−71	53	67	−15	−71	49	624
		R	21	−67	48	782	15	−71	53	58
Angular gyrus	40	L	−41	−38	39	63	−49	−48	45	104
		R	37	−45	45	64	46	−47	44	56
Inferior frontal sulcus	9/44	R	37	13	38	136				

The position of each area is given as the Talairach coordinates of the centre of mass of suprathreshold clusters ($p' < 10^{-3}$, corrected) of the group analysis. Size indicates number of voxels.

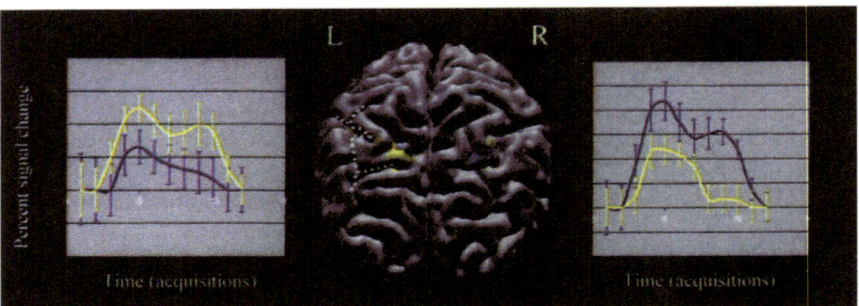

Figure 2. Multisubject GLM contrast maps ($p' < 10^{-3}$, corrected) superimposed on a 3-D reconstruction of the cortical surface of an individual normalised 3-D anatomy from the second block-design
study (Trojano et al., 2002). The figure (posterior view, left hemisphere on left side) shows the relative
contribution (for an explanation see caption to Figure 1) map between the coordinate (in blue) and the
categorical (in yellow) spatial tasks. The coordinate task produced a higher activation in the right PPC;
the categorical task activated mainly the left PPC. Other foci of activation are present in the both angular
gyrus bilaterally for both tasks and in the right prefrontal cortex for the coordinate task. As in the
previous experiment (see Figure 1), no imagery-related activation was observed in occipitotemporal
areas. The white dotted line corresponds to the intraparietal sulcus and its main branches.

The BOLD signal time courses from all the activated voxels in the PPC of each hemisphere,
averaged across subjects and epochs, are shown on the respective side of the map (note that BOLD
signal is plotted with different scales). On the left PPC the averaged signal time course reveals a
higher percentage signal change in the categorical task (yellow line) than in the coordinate task (blue
line); a reverse pattern is observed on the right side. Reprinted with permission of Elsevier Science
(Trojano et al., 2002).

activation induced by the *categorical* task produced a larger cluster size on the
left side. Moreover, the *coordinate* task specifically induced activation of the
right prefrontal cortex encroaching upon the posterior end of the inferior frontal
sulcus.

The analysis of single subjects' activations confirmed the robust finding that
the superior parietal lobules were engaged in both spatial imagery tasks.
Moreover, within the superior parietal lobules, four out of seven subjects
showed larger left hemisphere activation in the categorical task than in the
coordinate task, and five out of seven subjects showed larger right hemisphere
activation in the coordinate task than in the categorical task. Considering the
whole parietal lobes, the total number of activated voxels did not differ between
the two hemispheres (left parietal lobe: 4786 ± 1984; right parietal lobe: 3852 ±
1931; Wilcoxon $Z = 1.16$, $p = .24$) or between the two tasks (coordinate task:
5268 ± 2041; categorical task: 3369 ± 2262; Wilcoxon $Z = 1.54$, $p = .12$) across
the seven subjects; the mean percentage number of activated voxels did not
differ between the two tasks in the left parietal lobe (coordinate task: 46.3;
categorical task: 53.7; Wilcoxon $Z = 0.17$, $p = .87$), while it was significantly

higher in the coordinate task (73.7) than in the categorical task (26.3) in the right parietal lobe (Wilcoxon $Z = 2.03$, $p = .04$).

These findings confirmed that parietal lobes are strongly involved in the processing of spatially coded material in the imagery domain. Moreover, data pointed to a differential functional involvement of interconnected neural networks according to cognitive requirements of different spatial tasks. The coordinate judgement specifically relied on the activation of the right prefrontal cortex. In studies on visual and spatial mental imagery coactivation of frontal and parietal areas has often been reported and related to image generation or to image maintenance (Ishai, Ungerleider, & Haxby, 2000; Mellet, Petit, Mazoyer, Denis, & Tzourio, 1998; Thompson & Kosslyn, 2000). Since behavioural results of our experiment demonstrate that the categorical and the coordinate imagery tasks had equivalent processing load, the differential activation of right prefrontal cortex could be explained by a higher processing load on spatial working memory during the coordinate task (Smith & Jonides, 1999).

With respect to the issue of lateralisation of categorical and coordinate spatial judgements, Baciu, Koenig, Vernier, Bedoin, Rubin, and Segebarth (1999) showed a stronger activation of the left than of the right angular gyrus in a categorical task, and the reverse pattern of lateralisation in a coordinate task in the visual perception domain. Our findings are congruent with these data, but our whole-brain study allowed us to verify that some degree of relative lateralisation may also be found in regions other than the parietal cortex. In conclusion, the findings of this study support the idea that the superior parietal lobules are crucial for both categorical and coordinate spatial judgements. These regions, together with other parietal and prefrontal areas, showed a pattern of relative lateralisation, since the left hemisphere was more involved in the categorical task, while the coordinate task elicited activation of more extended regions of the right hemisphere and of right prefrontal regions thought to be involved in spatial working memory (Smith & Jonides, 1999). The involvement of a frontoparietal network in the processing of mental images has been confirmed by recent fMRI studies on both spatial (Knauff, Kassubek, Mulack, & Greenlee, 2000) and object (Ishai et al., 2000) imagery, but without any clear evidence of hemispheric asymmetry.

IS IT POSSIBLE TO DIFFERENTIATE THE ROLE OF SINGLE NEURAL STRUCTURES IN DIFFERENT COGNITIVE COMPONENTS OF SPATIAL MENTAL IMAGERY?

In functional neuroimaging like in psychometric studies (Michimata, 1997), it has to be considered that the observed differences in cortical activation might originate at different stages of the cognitive processes involved in the tasks. For example, it could be argued that the requirement of the coordinate judgement would elicit an image generation process more heavily dependent on the precise metric assembly of multi-part mental images, whereas the categorical judgement could induce a global, sketchier reconstruction of mental images. Alternatively, it could be hypothesised that generating a multipart mental image requires a metric spatially organised arrangement of its constituents, a cognitive step common to the two imagery tasks, and that the observed differences in cortical activation could arise during different spatial computations required by the categorical or the coordinate judgement. Novel experimental paradigms would be necessary to differentiate among the possible theoretical explanations of our findings. For instance, the coordinate/categorical distinction could be assessed in an experimental set including also two parallel visual perceptual conditions for the categorical and the coordinate judgement. However, this would imply several methodological drawbacks, since such perceptual tasks would be considerably easier than the imagery conditions, as has been stated in previous studies (French & Painter, 1991). Other experimental approaches, for example by means of event-related fMRI paradigms, will be necessary to determine which cortical regions are involved in the generation of mental images, and which in subsequent spatial judgements.

Thompson and Kosslyn (2000) propose four types of imagery processing: image generation, image inspection, image maintenance, and image transformation. Most imagery tasks probably involve more than one if not all of these. Furthermore, some degree of sequential processing will also be required. In the case of the mental clock task, e.g., it can be argued that first an image of an analogue clock has to be generated on the basis of the information about the first time. This image has to be maintained while the second image is generated on the basis of the second time, then both images are inspected and compared, which might involve some spatial transformation of the images. Traditionally, the cortical representation of these components of the imagery system could only be probed in neuropsychological or functional neuroimaging studies by the comparison of different imagery tasks requiring a different contribution from these components. With the development of techniques for event-related fMRI, however, it has become possible to investigate the representation of component cognitive processes in imagery (and many other cognitive areas) within one task, and often at the level of the single trial.

We applied event-related fMRI to the same task that had been studied with the classical block design in the studies reported above (Formisano et al., 2000, 2002; Linden et al., 2000). In this series of event-related fMRI experiments, the mental clock task was administered to six subjects altogether. The MR hardware was the same as above. We used a BOLD sensitive single shot EPI sequence (echo time, TE = 60 ms; flip angle, FA = 90°; matrix size = 64 × 64, voxel dimensions = 3 mm × 3 mm × 5 mm) that permitted whole-brain imaging (16 slices) in 1.6 s. Functional measurements were obtained every 2 s. Subjects again had to mentally construct analogue clocks from acoustically presented pairs of time and identify the greater angle while they kept the eyes open and directed on a fixation cross. Responses were indicated by button press with the right ($n = 3$) or left ($n = 3$) hand. Performance was again very good (95% correct trials), and the reaction time was around 3 s. Although the sampling rate was not much higher than the time required for the execution of the task (2 s vs. 3 s), the fairly stable interval between acoustic stimulation and button press response permitted the analysis of the sequence activation of the different cortical areas recruited for the task.

The first area to be activated was the auditory cortex (Figure 3A), followed by the dorsolateral prefrontal cortex (DLPFC), the posterior parietal cortex, the supplementary motor area, and, finally, the motor cortex contralateral to the hand used for the button press. While the DLPFC activation was present during the entire interval between auditory and motor cortex activation and no hemispheric difference could be observed, the posterior parietal activity showed two peaks that were clearly separated in time, with a cluster that was activated early during the task and shows a bilateral distribution (but left predominance) and a late cluster that was confined to the right PPC. The duration of activation of the early cluster and the onset of the late right cluster correlated with reaction time.

It has been suggested above that the mental clock task requires the formation, maintenance, and spatial manipulation of images. We would expect areas involved in image generation to show a relatively early onset of BOLD activation, while areas involved in image manipulation and comparison would become active later because they presume the completion of a neuronal process in the image generation areas. Areas involved in the maintenance of the mental images should show a rise of activation at about the same time as the image generation areas but, unlike these, stay active during the entire trial. Of the three regions that were found to differ in their temporal characteristics during execution of the mental clock task each matched the criteria for one of the imagery subsystems. The early posterior parietal cluster with a bilateral, but predominantly left, distribution can be regarded as responsible for image generation. The DLPFC was active during the entire delay interval and thus matches the criteria for the image maintenance area, which is compatible with the well-known role of this area in the maintenance of visual information (Munk et al., 2002). The right posterior parietal cortex was activated last, which indicates its role in the spatial manipulation and analysis of the images. This result is in keeping with the large body of neuropsychological and neuroimaging literature that has indicated the particular importance of the right posterior parietal cortex for visuospatial processing, particularly when precise metric judgements are required or when analysis of local features of imagined visual objects is required (Ishai, Ungerleider, & Haxby, 2002).

The present study, which was, to our knowledge, the first event-related functional neuroimaging study of mental imagery, could not address all aspects of the cerebral localisation of the subsystems of visuospatial imagery and their chronometry. In particular, the relationship of image inspection and spatial

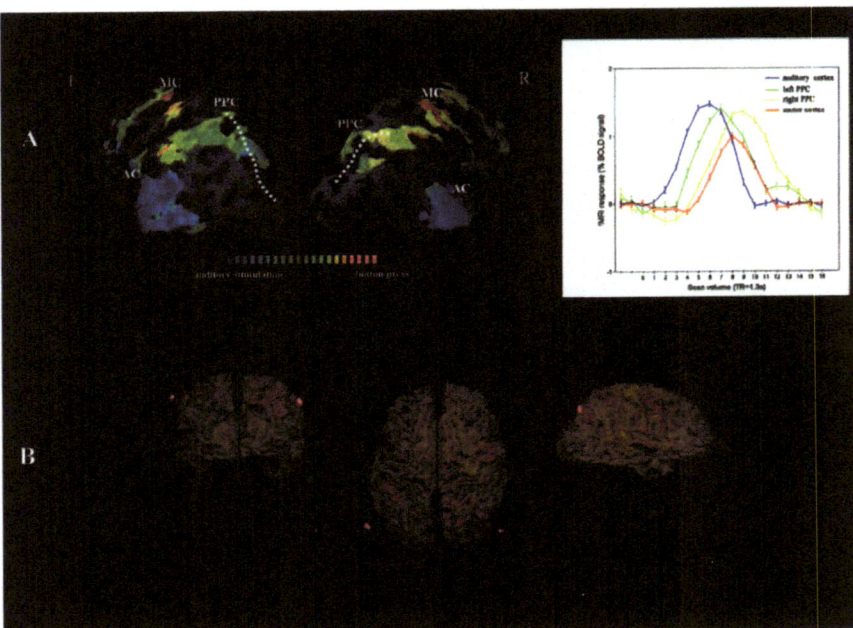

Figure 3. (A) Time-resolved multiple regression analysis of event-related fMRI time series. On the left, multisubject ($n = 6$) general linear model surface maps were superimposed on an inflated (lateral view) representation of the cortical sheet of a template brain normalised in Talairach space. The colour of significantly task-related voxels ($p' < .001$, corrected) encodes the latency of BOLD activation following the auditory presentation of the stimulus. Blue (red) colour indicates early (late) latencies of task-related activation corresponding to the auditory stimulation (motor response). Intermediate latencies of task-related activation are linearly represented according to the colour bar (Formisano et al., 2002). Dotted line indicates the intraparietal sulcus (posterior branch), PPC = posterior parietal cortex, AC = auditory cortex, PFC = prefrontal cortex, MC = motor cortex.

On the right, event-related BOLD responses of the auditory cortex, of the left and right posterior parietal cortex, and of the motor cortex during the execution of a single trial of the mental clock task. Reprinted with permission of Cell Press (Formisano et al., 2002).

(B) Head and cortex reconstruction from an anatomical MR data set of a single subject that shows the positions of the coil for rTMS (repetitive transcranial magnetic stimulation) stimulation in the left and right PPC. The rTMS coil was placed in correspondence of positions P3 and P4 of the international 10–20 EEG system. These positions were also marked using MR-visible vitamin E capsules (red spots on the skull) such that the relative displacement between fMRI activation in the PPC and sites of rTMS stimulation could be verified in individual subjects (see Sack et al., 2002).

analysis could not be clarified because, as in the previous block design studies, no significant activation of occipital and inferior temporal activation was observed during the mental clock task. The absence of imagery-related activation in early visual areas confirms the recent findings that certain imagery conditions, particularly those that rely on abstract patterns and schematic figures, produce activity in primary visual areas only to a small extent (Goebel et al., 1998a), or not at all (Mellet et al., 1996).

For a better differentiation of the image inspection and spatial transformation mechanisms, the design of paradigms requiring the detailed analysis of a mental image and its subsequent spatial manipulation might be useful. For these and related questions the further development and refinement of the appropriate MR hardware, fast MR sequences, and analytical tools for event-related and single-trial fMRI techniques will be pivotal.

The functional relevance of PPC activity during the mental clock task was investigated by a further study (Sack et al., 2002) that combined functional neuroimaging with unilateral repetitive transcranial magnetic stimulation (rTMS). This study confirmed that visuospatial operations are associated with activation of the intraparietal sulcus bilaterally, but showed that only rTMS to the right parietal lobe induced an impairment of performance (Figure 3B). This functional parietal asymmetry in processing spatial mental images might indicate a capacity of the right parietal lobe to compensate for a lesion of the left. Such an explanation would be compatible with the current theories on spatial hemineglect that implicate an asymmetrical distribution of spatial attention (Mesulam, 1999). According to such models, the left hemisphere shifts attention in a contraversive direction while the right hemisphere directs attention in both directions (thus participating in a bilateral attentional network for the right hemispace); a lesion of the right hemispheric attention network would lead to hemineglect for the left hemispace, whereas a corresponding left hemispheric lesion could be compensated for by the preserved (right) hemisphere, which also covers the contralesional (right) hemispace.

CONCLUSION

The set of studies reviewed here converge to demonstrate that cortical areas in the PPC, along the intraparietal sulcus, are robustly involved in spatial mental imagery and in other tasks requiring spatial transformations. PPC is bilaterally involved in different kinds of spatial judgement. Yet the degree to which right and left PPC are activated in different tasks is a function of task requirements. From event-related fMRI data we obtained evidence that left and right PPC are activated asynchronously during the clock task and this could reflect their different functional role in subserving cognitive components of visuospatial imagery.

PrEview proof published online May 2004

REFERENCES

Alivisatos, B., & Petrides, M. (1997). Functional activation of the human brain during mental rotation. *Neuropsychologia, 35,* 111–118.

Baciu, M., Koenig, O., Vernier, M. P., Bedoin, N., Rubin, C., & Segebarth, C. (1999). Categorical and coordinate spatial relations: fMRI evidence for hemispheric specialization. *Neuroreport, 10,* 1373–1378.

Brown, H. D., & Kosslyn, S. M. (1993). Cerebral lateralization. *Current Opinion in Neurobiology, 3*, 183–186.

Cabeza, R., & Nyberg, L. (2000). Imaging cognition II: An empirical review of 275 PET and fMRI studies. *Journal of Cognitive Neuroscience, 12*, 1–47.

Cohen, M. S., Kosslyn, S. M., Breiter, H. C., DiGirolamo, G. J., Thompson, W. L., Anderson, A. K., Brookheimer, S. Y., Rosen, B. R., & Belliveau, J. W. (1996). Changes in cortical activity during mental rotation: A mapping study using functional MRI. *Brain, 119*, 89–100.

Di Salle, F., Formisano, E., Linden, D. E. J., Goebel, R., Bonavita, S., Pepino, A., Smaltino, F., & Tedeschi, G. (1999). Exploring brain function with magnetic resonance imaging. *European Journal of Radiology, 30*, 84–94.

Farah, M. J., Hammond, K. M., Levine, D. N., & Calvanio, R. (1988). Visual and spatial imagery: Dissociable systems of representation. *Cognitive Psychology, 20*, 439–462.

Formisano, E., Di Salle, F., Linden, D. E. J., Trojano, L., Grossi, D., Zanella, F. E., & Goebel, R. (2000). Event-related fMRI during behaviorally controlled visuospatial imagery. *NeuroImage, 11*, S87.

Formisano, E., Linden, D. E. J., Di Salle, F., Trojano, L., Esposito, F., Sack, A. T., Grossi, D., Zanella, F. E., & Goebel, R. (2002). Tracking the mind's image in the brain. I: Time-resolved fMRI during visuospatial mental imagery. *Neuron, 35*, 185–194.

French, C. C., & Painter, J. (1991). Spatial processing of images and hemisphere function. *Cortex, 27*, 511–520.

Ghaem, O., Mellet, E., Crivello, F., Tzourio, N., Mazoyer, B., Berthoz, A., & Denis, M. (1997). Mental navigation along memorized routes activates the hippocampus, precuneus, and insula. *Neuroreport, 8*, 739–744.

Goebel, R., Khorram-Sefat, D., Muckli, L., Hacker, H., & Singer, W. (1998a). The constructive nature of vision: Direct evidence from functional magnetic resonance imaging studies of apparent motion and motion imagery. *European Journal of Neuroscience, 10*, 1563–1573.

Goebel, R., Linden, D. E. J., Lanfermann, H., Zanella, F. E., & Singer, W. (1998b). Functional imaging of mirror and inverse reading reveals separate coactivated networks for oculomotion and spatial transformations. *Neuroreport, 9*, 713–719.

Goebel, R., & Singer, W. (1999). Cortical surface-based statistical analysis of functional magnetic resonance imaging data. *NeuroImage, 9*, S64.

Grossi, D., Angelini, R., Pecchinenda, A., & Pizzamiglio, L. (1993). Left imaginal neglect in heminattention: Experimental study with the o'clock test. *Behavioral Neurology, 6*, 155–158.

Grossi, D., Modafferi, A., Pelosi, L., & Trojano, L. (1989). On the different roles of the two cerebral hemispheres in mental imagery: The "O'Clock test" in two clinical cases. *Brain and Cognition, 10*, 18–27.

Ishai, A., Ungerleider, L. G., & Haxby, J. V. (2000). Distributed neural systems for the generation of visual images. *Neuron, 28*, 979–990.

Ishai, A., Ungerleider, L. G., & Haxby, J. V. (2002). Visual imagery of famous faces: Effects of memory and attention revealed by fMRI. *NeuroImage, 16*, S595.

Knauff, M., Kassubek, J., Mulack, T., & Greenlee, M. W. (2000). Cortical activation evoked by visual mental imagery as measured by fMRI. *Neuroreport, 11*, 3957–3962.

Kosslyn, S. M. (1987). Seeing and imaging in the cerebral hemispheres: A computational approach. *Psychological Review, 94*, 148–175.

Kosslyn, S. M. (1994). *Image and brain*. Cambridge, MA: MIT Press.

Kosslyn, S. M., DiGirolamo, G. J., Thompson, W. L., & Alpert, N. M. (1998). Mental rotation of objects versus hands: Neural mechanisms revealed by positron emission tomography. *Psychophysiology, 3*, 151–161.

Kosslyn, S. M., Maljkovic, V., Hamilton, S. E., Horwitz, G., & Thompson, W. L. (1995). Two types of image generation: Evidence for left and right hemisphere processes. *Neuropsychologia, 33*, 1485–1510.

Kosslyn, S. M., & Sussmann, A. L. (1995). Roles of imagery in perception: Or, there is no such thing as immaculate perception. In M. Gazzaniga (Ed.), *The cognitive neurosciences* (pp. 1035–1042). Cambridge, MA: MIT Press.

Levine, D. N., Warach, J., & Farah, M. (1985). Two visual systems in mental imagery: Dissociation of "what" and "where" in imagery disorders due to bilateral posterior cerebral lesions. *Neurology, 35,* 1010–1018.

Linden, D. E. J. (2002). Five hundred years of brain images. *Archives of Neurology, 59,* 308–313.

Linden, D. E. J., Formisano, E., Di Salle, F., Trojano, L., Zanella, F. E., Steinmetz, H., & Goebel, R. (2000). Tracking the mind's image in the brain: Single trial fMRI during behaviourally controlled visuospatial imagery. *European Journal of Neuroscience, 12*(Suppl. 11), 86c.

Linden, D. E. J., Prvulovic, D., Formisano, E., Völlinger, M., Zanella, F. E., Goebel, R., & Dierks, T. (1999). The functional neuroanatomy of target detection: An fMRI study of visual and auditory oddball tasks. *Cerebral Cortex, 9,* 815–823.

Luzzatti, C., Vecchi, T., Agazzi, D., Cesa-Bianchi, M., & Vergani, C. (1998). A neurological dissociation between preserved visual and impaired spatial processing in mental imagery. *Cortex, 34,* 461–469.

Malach, R., Reppas, J. B., Benson, R. R., Kwong, K. K., Jiang, H., Kennedy, W. A., Ledden, P. J., Brady, T. J., Rosen, B. R., & Tootell, R. B. (1995). Object-related activity revealed by functional magnetic resonance imaging in human occipital cortex. *Proceedings of the National Academy of Sciences, USA, 92,* 8135–8139.

Mellet, E., Petit, L., Mazoyer, B., Denis, M., & Tzourio, N. (1998). Reopening the mental imagery debate: Lessons from functional anatomy. *Neuroimage, 8,* 129–139.

Mellet, E., Tzourio, N., Crivello, F., Joliot, M., Denis, M., & Mazoyer, B. (1996). Functional anatomy of spatial mental imagery generated from verbal instructions. *Journal of Neuroscience, 16,* 6504–6512.

Mellet, E., Tzourio, N., Denis, M., & Mazoyer, B. (1995). A positron emission tomography of visual and mental spatial exploration. *Journal of Cognitive Neuroscience, 7,* 433–445.

Mesulam, M. M. (1999). Spatial attention and neglect: Parietal, frontal and cingulate contributions to the mental representation and attentional targeting of salient extrapersonal events. *Philosophical Transactions of the Royal Society of London: Biological Sciences, 354,* 1325–1346.

Michimata, C. (1997). Hemispheric processing of categorical and coordinate spatial relations in vision and visual imagery. *Brain and Cognition, 33,* 370–387.

Milner, A. D., & Goodale, M. A. (1995). *The visual brain in action.* Oxford, UK: Oxford University Press.

Munk, M. H. J., Linden, D. E. J., Muckli, L., Lanfermann, H., Zanella, F. E., Singer, W., & Goebel R. (2002). Distributed cortical systems in visual short-term memory revealed by event-related functional magnetic resonance imaging. *Cerebral Cortex, 12,* 866–876.

O'Craven, K. M., & Kanwisher, N. (2000). Mental imagery of faces and places activates corresponding stimulus-specific brain regions. *Journal of Cognitive Neuroscience, 12,* 1013–1023.

Paivio, A. (1978). Comparisons of mental clocks. *Journal of Experimental Psychology: Human Perception, 4,* 61–71.

Sack, A. T., Sperling, J. M., Prvulovic, D., Formisano, E., Goebel, R., Di Salle, F., Dierks, T., & Linden, D. E. J. (2002). Tracking the mind's image in the brain. II: Transcranial magnetic stimulation reveals parietal asymmetry in visuospatial imagery. *Neuron, 35,* 195–204.

Sathian, K., Zangaladze, A., Hoffmann, J. M., & Grafton, S. T. (1997). Feeling with the mind's eye. *Neuroreport, 8,* 3877–3881.

Smith, E. E., & Jonides, J. (1999). Storage and executive processes in the frontal lobes. *Science, 283,* 1657–1661.

Thompson, W. L., & Kosslyn, S. M. (2000). Neural systems activated during visual mental imagery—a review and meta-analysis. In A. W. Toga & J. C. Mazziotta (Eds.), *Brain mapping: The systems* (pp. 535–560). San Diego: Academic Press.

Trojano, L., & Grossi, D. (1994). A critical review of mental imagery defects. *Brain and Cognition*, *24*, 213–243.

Trojano, L., Grossi, D., Linden, D. E. J., Formisano, E., Goebel, R., Cirillo, S., Elefante, R., & Di Salle, F. (2002). Coordinate and categorical judgements in spatial imagery: An fMRI study. *Neuropsychologia, 40*, 1666–1674.

Trojano, L., Grossi, D., Linden, D. E. J., Formisano, E., Hacker, H., Zanella, F. E., Goebel, R., & Di Salle, F. (2000). Matching two imagined clocks: The functional anatomy of spatial analysis in the absence of visual stimulation. *Cerebral Cortex, 10*, 473–481.

Ungerleider, L. G., & Haxby, J. V. (1994). "What" and "where" in the human brain. *Current Opinions in Neurobiology, 4*, 157–165.

Ungerleider, L. G., & Mishkin, M. (1982). Two cortical visual systems. In D. J. Ingle, M. A. Goodale, & R. J. W. Mansfield (Eds.), *Analysis of visual behavior* (pp. 549–586). Cambridge, MA: MIT Press.

EUROPEAN JOURNAL OF COGNITIVE PSYCHOLOGY, 2004, *16* (5), 673–695

A PET meta-analysis of object and spatial mental imagery

Angélique Mazard, Nathalie Tzourio-Mazoyer, Fabrice Crivello, Bernard Mazoyer, and Emmanuel Mellet

Groupe d'Imagerie Neurofonctionnelle, CNRS, CEA, Université de Caen and Université René-Descartes, France

Neuroimaging studies have described the functional neuroanatomy of mental imagery. Taken separately, specific studies vary in the nature of the task used and are limited by statistical power and sensitivity. We took advantage of a multistudy PET database of 54 subjects acquired in our laboratory to reveal the neural bases of spatial versus object mental imagery tasks. Our first goal was to evaluate to what extent the activated foci elicited by both object and spatial studies overlap. A second aim was to compare activations elicited by spatial imagery tasks to those elicited by object imagery tasks. We also explored applying regression analyses to the relationships between the scores on the Mental Rotations Test (MRT) and changes in regional cerebral blood flow (rCBF) during spatial and object imagery tasks. This meta-analysis yielded the following observations: (1) both spatial and object imagery tasks shared a common neural network composed of occipitotemporal (ventral pathway) and occipitoparietal (dorsal pathway) regions and also by a set of frontal regions (related to memory); (2) the superior parietal cortex was more strongly implicated during spatial imagery; (3) object imagery specifically engaged the anterior part of the ventral pathway, including the fusiform, parahippocampal, and hippocampal gyrus; (4) object imagery activated the early visual cortex, whereas spatial imagery induced a deactivation of the early visual cortex; (5) blood flow values in some of the regions noted above were positively correlated with scores on the MRT: the higher the subjects performed on the MRT, the more pronounced the rCBF was in these regions. These results may reconcile some of the apparent discrepancies among previous studies concerning the activation of early visual cortex in mental imagery. They also contribute to a better knowledge of the neural bases of object and spatial mental imagery.

Correspondence should be addressed to Emmanuel Mellet, Groupe d'Imagerie Neurofonction-nelle, GIP Cyceron, Bvd H. Becquerel, BP 5229, 14074 CAEN Cedex, France.
Email: mellet@cyceron.fr
Angélique Mazard was supported by the Fondation pour la Recherche Médicale.
The authors are grateful to Catharine Mason and Alan Young for grammatical corrections of the manuscript.

http://www.tandf.co.uk/journals/pp/09541446.html   DOI: 10.1080/09541440340000484

It is now well established that both visual mental imagery and visual perception rely on sets of distinct subsystems (Farah, 1984; Kosslyn, 1994). A major concern of neuroimaging studies that identified the cerebral bases of visual imagery has been to assess the extent to which visual imagery and visual perception share common cerebral structures (Kosslyn et al., 1993; Kosslyn, Thompson, & Alpert, 1997; Mellet, Tzourio, Denis, & Mazoyer, 1995). In agreement with the theoretical framework proposed by Kosslyn (1987, 1994), it has been established that both visual perception and visual imagery rely on a "what" and "where" functional dichotomy (see Mellet, Petit, Mazoyer, Denis, & Tzourio, 1998, for a review). According to this dichotomy, figurative aspects of both mental images and visual percepts are processed along the ventral occipitotemporal route while the dorsal occipitoparietal route processes the spatial features. Note, however, that this distinction is not absolute since most of the neuroimaging studies that dealt with spatial imagery tasks not only reported dorsal activation but also activation along the ventral route. In the same vein, studies that focused on figurative imagery reported occipitoparietal activation together with the activation in the ventral pathway (Ishai, Ungerleider, & Haxby, 2000; Lambert, Sampaio, Scheiber, & Mauss, 2002).

In addition to these uncontroversial findings, divergent neuroimaging results were reported regarding the involvement of the early visual cortex (Brodmann Areas 17–18), within and around the calcarine fissure, during visual mental imagery. Some researchers have reported activation of the early visual cortex, whereas others have not (see Roland & Gulyas, 1994, for reviews; Kosslyn, Ganis, & Thompson, 2001; Kosslyn & Ochsner, 1994; Mellet et al., 1998; Sakai & Miyashita, 1994). These discrepancies have questioned some aspects of Kosslyn's model since the early visual cortex had been proposed to be a key part of the neural substrate of the so-called visual buffer (Kosslyn, 1994). This buffer would be shared by both perception and imagery and is thought to implement a topographic representation of either a perceptual or a mental image. Various factors have been considered in the neuroimaging literature in order to explain these divergent reports: the nature of the baseline condition, the level of resolution of mental images and the type of neuroimaging techniques used (i.e., positron emission tomography, PET, or functional magnetic resonance imaging, fMRI), but no definite explanation has emerged. In the present paper we consider another alternative account, which is related to the spatial or object nature of the mental imagery task. Indeed, most studies dealing with spatial imagery have not reported early visual cortex activation whereas, in those studies in which an activation was noted, figurative imagery tasks were employed (Kosslyn et al., 2001; Thompson, Kosslyn, Sukel, & Alpert, 2001).

In the present paper, we report new analyses of PET data collected in our laboratory including nine mental imagery conditions, 54 subjects, and a total of 323 scans. The aim of this meta-analysis was two-fold. First, we wanted to discover which brain regions are activated during visual mental imagery in general, whatever the nature of the imagery task. In the framework of the imagery debate, the large number of scans and subjects included in this analysis offers better sensitivity to small effects and allows one to detect even small activation of the early visual cortex. Our second goal was to compare two kinds of imagery tasks: tasks that mainly dealt with the spatial properties of the mental image, such as mental scanning or mental navigation, and those that required the subjects to imagine colour, shape, and texture of objects. This comparison will highlight the brain areas that are either specific to a given modality (i.e., spatial or figurative) or that are significantly more activated in one modality than in the other. Finally individual differences in imagery ability could also be partly responsible for the discrepancies in the literature. Adopting an exploratory approach, we investigated whether the individual ability for mental imagery, as assessed by the Mental Rotations Test (MRT; Vandenberg & Kuse, 1978), could explain the interindividual variability of regional blood flow increases during the mental imagery tasks.

MATERIALS AND METHODS

Experimental design

The data from nine mental imagery conditions were analysed with a multistudy statistical model. We distinguished two categories of mental imagery tasks in this analysis: the first included the tasks that relied on spatial properties of images, and the second comprised those that included a strong object component. More specifically, the spatial imagery tasks included mental scanning, mental navigation, or spatial construction. The object imagery tasks required the subjects to retrieve a representation of figurative attributes of the stimuli (e.g., shape, configuration). The nine imagery conditions are detailed below. Among the nine conditions, we have classified seven of them as spatial imagery conditions and two of them as object imagery conditions.

All conditions were conducted with eyes closed in total darkness; a black and opaque chamber covered the whole PET camera. All conditions except one (baseline condition of Study 6) were compared to a rest condition. During this rest condition, subjects were instructed to keep their eyes closed, to relax, to refrain from moving, and to avoid any structured mental activity such as counting or rehearsing. This condition has been widely used as a basic control condition in our laboratory (Mazoyer et al., 2001). It has recently been proposed as a good "baseline" physiological state (Gusnard & Raichle, 2001).

Spatial imagery conditions

Condition 1. Mental exploration (Mellet et al., 1995). Seven right-handed healthy male French students participated in this study. Normalised regional cerebral blood flow (NrCBF) was measured four times for each subject, replicating a series of two conditions: mental exploration of an island map and rest in total darkness. For the mental exploration condition, the subjects were instructed to generate a mental image of a map of an island that they had previously visually explored; six landmarks were located on the periphery of the island. Then, they were asked to explore this mental map according to the following instructions: "Starting from the northern extremity of the island and following its periphery, you have to move mentally clockwise from landmark to landmark, pausing a few seconds on each one; after completing the clockwise exploration in about 40 s, you have to explore it again in a counterclockwise direction at the same speed."

Condition 2. Spatial mental construction (Mellet, Tzourio, Crivello, Joliot, Denis, & Mazoyer, 1996).   Nine right-handed healthy male French students took part in this study. We obtained four sequential PET measurements of the NrCBF of each subject, replicating a series of two experimental conditions: a spatial mental construction task and a rest condition. During the mental construction task the subjects were requested to build four three-dimensional (3-D) mental objects made out of twelve cubes (Shepard & Metzler, 1971). The task itself consisted first in visualising one cube, which served as the starting point of the construction, and then adding eleven other cubes according to a list of directional words given verbally through earphones at 0.5 Hz. The lists were randomly generated using the six directional French words: "haut" ("up"), "bas" ("down"), "droite" ("right"), "gauche" ("left"), "avant" ("front"), "arrière" ("back"). At the end of the mental construction of the object, the subjects had to visualise the entire object during 5 s, and then delete it from their mind before visualising again the starting cube and building the next object from another list of directional words.

Condition 3. Mental navigation (Ghaëm et al., 1997).   Five right-handed healthy male French students participated in this study. Four sequential measurements of the NrCBF were obtained from each subject, replicating a series of two experimental conditions: a rest condition and a mental navigation task. The day before the PET scanning, the subjects walked within an environment (a park) they had never seen before and were instructed to memorise key landmarks. The mental navigation task performed in the PET camera consisted of mentally recalling the visual and sensory-motor mental images of their walk from a route perspective, following the path between two named landmarks, and pressing a key when the second landmark was reached. Five different segments, randomly presented, were used during each replication of the mental navigation condition.

Condition 4. Mental scanning (Mellet et al., 2000a).   Six right-handed healthy male French students took part in this study. Four to six sequential measurements of NrCBF were obtained from each subject, replicating two or three times a series of two experimental conditions (because of technical problems, the PET camera did not start during part of the acquisition resulting in missing replications for some subjects). The two experimental conditions were rest and mental scanning of a map. During the mental map task, subjects were asked to keep eyes closed and to visualise a previously memorised map that included seven coloured dots. They were then given the name of two coloured dots (e.g., "red", "blue") through earphones and had to imagine a laser dot following the path segment drawn on the original map between the two dots. Once the second dot was reached, the subjects had to press a button with their right index finger—after they performed this action, the names of a second pair of dots were presented auditorily.

Condition 5. Mental scanning of verbally described environments (Mellet, Bricogne, Crivello, Mazoyer, Denis, & Tzourio-Mazoyer, 2002). This condition is similar to Condition 4 except that the mental map was mentally built after the subjects read a descriptive text. Six right-handed healthy male French students participated in this study. Eight measurements of NrCBF were obtained from each subject, replicating four times a series of two experimental conditions: a mental scanning task of verbally described environments and a rest condition. In this study, two different texts describing distinct environments (a leisure park and a town) were adapted from the study of Taylor and Tversky (1992). The texts described the environment from a survey perspective (i.e., using the canonical terms "north", "south", "east", and "west"). During mental scanning, the subjects closed their eyes and were told to visualise the environment as accurately as possible. They were then given (through earphones) the names of two landmarks (e.g., "church", "school") and were to imagine a laser dot following the path segment between the two landmarks. Once the second landmark was reached, the subjects had to press a button with their right index finger—after they performed this action, the names of a second pair of landmarks were presented auditorily.

Condition 6. High-resolution mental imagery based on visual or verbal descriptions (Mellet, Tzourio-Mazoyer, Bricogne, Mazoyer, Kosslyn, & Denis, 2000b). Seven right-handed healthy male French students participated in this study. There were three PET conditions: imagery after visual learning (6a), imagery after verbal learning (6b), and a baseline condition. For the two mental imagery conditions, the subjects memorised two scenes during the 15 min prior to scanning. In the visual learning condition, the subjects were asked to study and memorise scenes. In the verbal learning condition, the subjects were instructed to listen to verbal descriptions of how shapes were to be arranged and to form and memorise a visual image for each of the described scenes. Each scene was composed of four simple geometric shapes, arranged on a base; the scenes differed only in the ordering of the elements on the base. During the PET measurements, the subjects performed the imagery task, whatever the modality of learning, with the cues and comparison statements being delivered through earphones. Each condition consisted of nine comparison statements, alternating from one scene to the other. The comparison statements required the subjects to evaluate the relative height of the scene over two named points; the differences were subtle, and hence high resolution was required. The subjects had to respond by saying "right" or "wrong" into a microphone connected to a computer. After each response, the computer recorded the response time and then 750 ms later delivered the identification number of the next scene. Another 4 s later, a new comparison statement was delivered. Both imagery conditions (6a and 6b) were compared to a baseline task. During the baseline task, the subjects closed their eyes, listened to randomly chosen comparison statements delivered every 7 s, and alternatively said "right" and "wrong" after each term.

Condition 7. High-resolution mental imagery with different noise environments (Mazard, Mazoyer, Etard, Tzourio-Mazoyer, Kosslyn, & Mellet, 2002). Six right-handed healthy male French students took part in this study. This task was adapted from that used in the study just summarised (Mellet et al., 2000b). In the mental imagery task, subjects were asked to memorise 3-D sets of geometric forms on a base, which were presented visually, and then to judge subtle aspects of the scenes. In addition, we tested the effect of the "fMRI-like" noise environment on the mental imagery task. The sound produced by a clinical EPI-BOLD sequence was recorded using a nonmagnetic microphone near the radio frequency head coil (GE sigma 1.5T; TR = 6 s; TE = 60 ms; FA = 90 s). We monitored NrCBF in four different conditions. Two conditions were performed in a silent "PET-like" environment: a mental imagery task (7a) and a rest condition. During the other two conditions, the "fMRI-like" noise was played back from a digital audio tape and delivered through loudspeakers in the PET room. The remaining two conditions were a mental imagery task (7b) and a rest condition. All conditions were replicated twice in five subjects and once in one subject.

Object imagery conditions

Condition 8. Mental imagery of landmarks (Ghaëm et al., 1997). Five right-handed healthy male French students participated in this study. Four sequential measurements of NrCBF were obtained from each subject, replicating a series of two experimental conditions: a rest condition and static visual imagery of landmarks. The day before PET scanning, subjects walked within an environment (a park) they had never seen before and had to memorise key landmarks. During the static visual imagery task, subjects were instructed to visualise a landmark upon hearing its name through earphones and to maintain its mental image until they heard another landmark name 10 s later.

Condition 9. Mental imagery from concrete word definitions versus rest (Mellet, Tzourio, Denis, & Mazoyer, 1998).   Eight right-handed healthy male French students took part in this study. Six sequential measurements of NrCBF were obtained from each subject, replicating a series of two experimental conditions three times: listening to the definition of a concrete word and generating the corresponding mental image, and a rest condition. In the imagery task, the subjects were instructed to listen attentively to and understand 15 words and their definitions, taken from a French dictionary, verbally delivered through earphones. Each word and its accompanying definition were read in 6 s, followed by 2 s of silence before the next stimulus was delivered. The task duration was 120 s, starting 30 s before and maintained during the 90 s of the PET data acquisition. The words delivered during the imagery condition were of common use and easy to associate with an image, referring to objects or animals (such as "bottle", "guitar", "lion"). The definitions described figural, physical, or functional features of the objects or the animals. The definitions were thus very likely to result in spontaneous visual mental imagery activity. In addition, in order to induce sustained mental imagery, the subjects were explicitly encouraged to produce visual images evoked by words and to modify or refine each image as they listened to the definition following the word.

Subjects

A total of 54 right-handed male French students (age 18–35 years old) were included in this meta-analysis. Five of them performed both an object imagery task and a spatial imagery task (Conditions 3 and 5). More precisely, 13 subjects performed an object imagery condition and 46 performed a spatial imagery condition. Handedness was assessed with the Edinburgh Inventory (Oldfield, 1971). All subjects were free from neurological disease or injury and had no abnormalities in their T1-weighted magnetic resonance images (MRI). Written informed consent was obtained from each subject after the procedures had been fully explained. The local ethics committee approved all studies included in our meta-analysis.

In order to ensure optimal homogeneity of the sample of subjects with respect to their imagery abilities, subjects were selected as high visuospatial imagers on the basis of their scores on the MRT (Vandenberg & Kuse, 1978); all subjects scored beyond the 50th percentile of a population of 120 male subjects. The mean test score for all subjects was 16.46 ± 2.16 (mean $\pm$ *SD*).

Imaging

Measurements of the normalised regional cerebral blood flow (NrCBF) were obtained from each subject on two different cameras: an ECAT 953B/31 PET camera for Conditions 1, 2, and 3 (time acquisition: 80 s); and an ECAT exact HR+ camera for the other six conditions (time acquisition: 90 s). A single scan was acquired and reconstructed (including a correction for head attenuation using a measured transmission scan) with a Hanning filter of 0.5 mm^{-1} cut off frequency and a pixel size of 2×2 mm^2. The time delay between scans was 8 min.

Data analysis

In order to be included in the analysis, all the 323 scans were processed using the same procedure. After automatic realignment (AIR; Woods, Grafton, Holmes, Cherry, & Mazziotta, 1998), the original brain images were transformed into the MNI (Montreal National Institute) space (Friston, Holmes, Poline, Frith, & Frackowiak, 1995). The images were smoothed using a Gaussian filter of 12 mm FWHM leading to a final smoothness of 15 mm FWHM. The rCBF was normalised within and between subjects using a proportional model.

SPM-99 software was used to compute a multistudy analysis using the general linear model. Simple comparisons within each condition focused on the differences between a mental imagery task versus a baseline (rest in eight conditions, nonrest in one condition). All comparisons within each condition and within each study were computed and then combined in a conjunction analysis. Because activation and baseline conditions differed across studies, the conjunction analysis appears to be the most suitable approach to reveal effects common to the nine imagery conditions (Price & Friston, 1997). Conjunctions imply that activations must be present in all contrasts (mental imagery minus baseline) in order to be detected and it is thus a conservative approach, which avoids false-positive activations. In addition, outlying values did not influence the results (Friston, Holmes, Price, Büchel, & Worsley, 1999). The corresponding activation map was thresholded at $p < .001$ confidence level (uncorrected for multiple comparisons). The voxel amplitude t-map was transformed to a Z volume.

We also computed a comparison between the two types of tasks: (spatial tasks minus baselines) minus (object tasks minus baselines). In order to avoid any artifactual activation in the comparison caused by a deactivation during object imagery as compared to baseline, voxels that were not significant at $p = .05$ (uncorrected) in the spatial imagery versus baseline contrasts were excluded by masking. This activation map highlighted activations that were specific to the spatial imagery conditions, or more important in these conditions than in the object imagery conditions at $p < .001$ (uncorrected for multiple comparisons). The same procedure was used to reveal the specific activation map during object imagery conditions at $p < .001$ (uncorrected for multiple comparisons), using the comparison: (object tasks minus baselines) minus (spatial tasks minus baselines).

In addition, we performed two reverse comparisons, to discover the deactivations specific to spatial and to object imagery conditions, respectively at

$p < .001$ (uncorrected for multiple comparisons). These comparisons were thus: (baselines minus spatial tasks) minus (baselines minus object tasks) and (baselines minus object tasks) minus (baselines minus spatial tasks).

Linear regressions were computed between the difference noted in the scans of NrCBF during each imagery condition as compared to its baseline and the MRT scores recorded for each subject. Two regressions were performed separately for spatial imagery and object imagery conditions. Regression maps were thresholded at $p < .001$ (uncorrected for multiple comparisons).

Anatomical localisation of the maximum Z-score relied on the automated anatomical labelling of activations in SPM using a macroscopic anatomical parcellation of the MNI MRI single subject brain (Tzourio-Mazoyer et al., 2002).

PET RESULTS

NrCBF increases: Conjunction of all the nine imagery conditions

(See Table 1 and Figure 1A.) This analysis revealed regions that were activated in all of the nine mental imagery conditions compared to their respective baseline conditions.

We found a widespread bilateral activation in the parietal lobe, including the intraparietal sulcus and the precuneus, extending to the right angular gyrus and to the left middle occipital gyrus. In addition, we detected several foci in the frontal lobe, including a bilateral activation in the depth of the superior frontal sulcus and an activation of the anterior part of the left superior frontal sulcus and of the right inferior frontal gyrus. Another focus of activation was detected in the right middle frontal gyrus. Activations were also evident in the left superior part of the temporal pole and bilaterally in the inferior temporal gyrus, belonging to the so-called ventral pathway. We also detected bilateral activation of the anterior insula and one focus of activation in the right anterior part of the anterior cingulate cortex. The cerebellar vermis was also activated. Note that this conjunction analysis did not reveal any activation of the early visual cortex.

Areas more activated in spatial imagery conditions than in object imagery conditions

(See Table 2 and Figure 1B.) These conditions elicited large bilateral activation of the entire superior part of the parietal lobe: the bilateral precuneus, extending to the bilateral superior parietal gyrus and the right superior occipital gyrus. The middle occipital gyrus was also activated. A focus of activation was observed in the right middle cingulate cortex. In the frontal lobe, blood flow increased in the left middle frontal gyrus and extended to the superior frontal gyrus.

TABLE 1
Conjunction analysis revealing foci of significant NrCBF increases common to all of the nine mental imagery conditions as compared to baseline (p < .001, uncorrected for multiple comparisons)

Anatomical location of max. voxel activation	Coordinates			
	x	y	z	Z-score
L. intraparietal sulcus	−22	−70	52	7.8
R. intraparietal sulcus/precuneus	32	−66	48	6.9
R. intraparietal sulcus/angular gyrus	42	−60	48	5.7
L. middle occipital gyrus/intraparietal sulcus	−32	−82	30	3.6
L. superior frontal sulcus	−28	0	56	6.8
L. middle cingulate cortex	−4	14	42	6.4
L. superior frontal gyrus	−16	8	48	5.7
R. superior frontal sulcus	36	−4	54	5.3
R. middle frontal gyrus	28	0	64	4.7
L. superior frontal sulcus—anterior part	−28	50	16	5.7
R. inferior frontal gyrus—orbital part	28	46	−18	5.3
R. middle frontal gyrus	44	38	22	4.7
R. middle frontal gyrus	42	44	16	4.4
L. superior temporal gyrus/temp. pole—sup. part	−62	4	−10	4.2
R. inferior temporal gyrus	72	−40	−16	4.9
L. inferior temporal gyrus	−60	−38	−16	3.9
L. anterior insula	−24	20	−4	6.2
R. anterior insula	30	16	−4	3.6
R. anterior cingulate cortex	10	36	12	3.5
Cerebellar vermis lobule IV–V	0	−58	−16	4.8
R. cerebellar vermis lobule IV–V	2	−50	−20	4.2
R. cerebellar vermis lobule I–II	6	−44	−24	4.1

The data are local maxima of activated region detected with SPM 99 software. The anatomical localisation of the maximum Z-scores of these regions is given on the basis of the MNI template, using their stereotactic coordinates in mm (R: right; L: left).

Figure 1 (opposite). **(A)** Left, right, and superior 3-D view rendering of the statistical map revealing the areas activated when subjects formed images compared to baseline conditions (conjunction analysis of spatial and object imagery, see Table 1). **(B)** Superior 3-D view rendering of the statistical map showing the areas activated when subjects formed spatial images compared to object conditions. Plots show the local maxima (ΔNrCBF as percentage of the baseline NrCBF value) during each imagery condition in the intraparietal sulcus (IPS, see Table 2). **(C)** Inferior 3-D view rendering of statistical map revealing the activation within the inferior temporal lobe when subjects formed object images compared to spatial conditions. Plots show the local maximum during each imagery condition in the inferior temporal lobe ($x = -44$, $y = -16$, $z = -26$; see Table 3). The Z-maps were thresholded at $Z = 3.09$ (p < .001; uncorrected for multiple comparison). Stereotactic coordinates of local maxima are given based on the MNI coordinates.

A

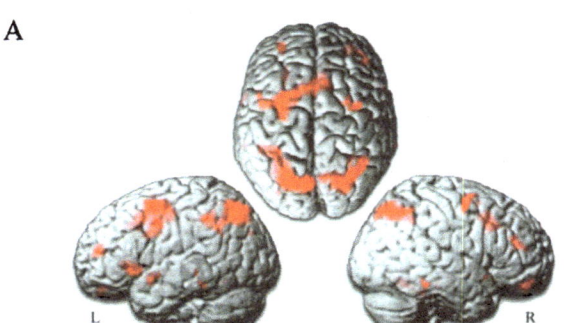

B

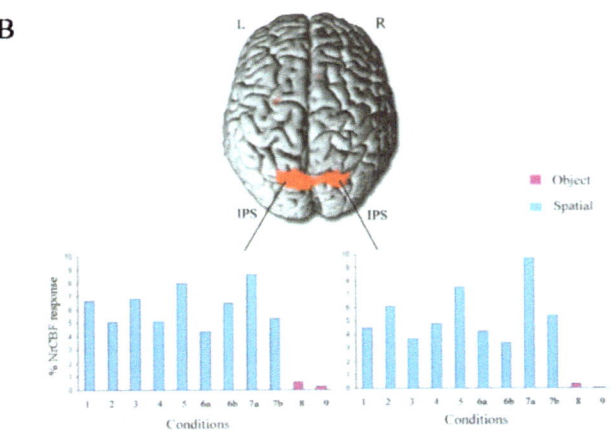

C

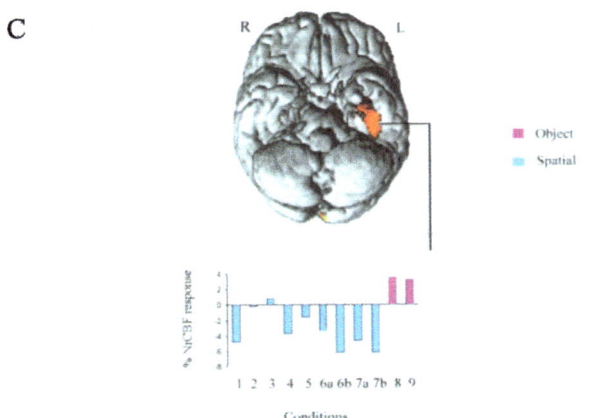

683

TABLE 2

Comparison analysis revealing foci of significant NrCBF increases between spatial imagery and object imagery (*p* < .001, uncorrected for multiple comparisons)

Anatomical location of max. voxel activation	Coordinates			
	x	*y*	*z*	Z-score
L. precuneus/superior parietal gyrus	−12	−70	46	>8.2
R. precuneus/superior parietal gyrus	18	−72	50	>8.2
R. superior occipital gyrus	32	−70	46	>8.2
R. middle occipital gyrus	40	−76	32	>8.2
R. middle cingulate cortex	8	18	38	7.6
L. middle/superior frontal gyrus	−28	−2	54	7.4

The data are local maxima of activated region detected with SPM 99 software. The anatomical localisation of the maximum Z-scores of these regions is given on the basis of the MNI template, using their stereotactic coordinates in mm (R: right; L: left).

TABLE 3

Comparison analysis revealing foci of significant NrCBF increases between object imagery and spatial imagery (*p* < .001, uncorrected for multiple comparisons)

Anatomical location of max. voxel activation	Coordinates			
	x	*y*	*z*	Z-score
L. Heschl's gyrus	−42	−20	8	5.6
L. superior temporal gyrus	−46	−24	14	5.3
R. Heschl's gyrus	40	−24	8	4.6
R. superior temporal gyrus	50	−24	10	4.3
L. inferior temporal gyrus/fusiform gyrus	−44	−16	−26	6.1
L. parahippocampal gyrus/hippocampus	−28	−10	−22	5.6
R. occipitotemporal junction	42	−50	−10	4.5
L. calcarine fissure	−2	−102	10	7.2
R. calcarine fissure	8	−88	12	4.7

The data are local maxima of activated region detected with SPM 99 software. The anatomical localisation of the maximum Z-scores of these regions is given on the basis of the MNI template, using their stereotactic coordinates in mm (R: right; L: left).

Areas more activated in object imagery conditions than in spatial imagery conditions

(See Table 3 and Figure 1C.) This comparison revealed that object imagery conditions induced a greater NrCBF increase in the temporal lobe, namely in the bilateral Heschl's gyrus extending to the superior temporal gyrus. Another focus

TABLE 4

Comparison analysis revealing foci of significant NrCBF decreases during spatial imagery ($p < .001$, uncorrected for multiple comparisons)

Anatomical location of max. voxel activation	Coordinates			
	x	y	z	Z-score
R. supramarginal gyrus/Rolandic operculum	58	−20	24	>8.2
L. calcarine fissure	−4	−100	10	7.2
L. cuneus/calcarine fissure	−2	−104	12	7.0
L. cuneus/superior occipital gyrus	−18	−100	12	6.0

The data are local maxima of deactivated region detected with SPM 99 software. The anatomical localisation of the maximum Z-scores of these regions is given on the basis of the MNI template, using their stereotactic coordinates in mm (R: right; L: left).

of activation was found in the posterior part of the right temporal lobe near its junction with the occipital lobe. In the left hemisphere, a cluster of activation spread to the inferior temporal gyrus, the parahippocampal gyrus and the hippocampus. This activation was specific to the object imagery conditions and this region was found to be deactivated in the spatial imagery conditions, as shown in Figure 1C. In the occipital lobe, two clusters of activated voxels were also detected within the calcarine fissure corresponding to primary visual area, as shown in Figure 2A.

Areas deactivated in spatial imagery conditions

(See Table 4 and Figure 2A.) A NrCBF decrease was observed in the right supramarginal gyrus near the right Rolandic operculum. In the occipital lobe, we found two foci of deactivation in the left cuneus near the superior occipital gyri. It is noteworthy that the calcarine fissure was found to be deactivated in these conditions. The calcarine cortex was thus deactivated in spatial imagery tasks whereas it was activated in object imagery tasks.

Areas deactivated in object imagery conditions

No cluster was identified in this analysis at $p < .001$ statistical threshold.

Regression analyses between MRT scores and CBF increases during the tasks

(See Table 5 and Figure 2B, C.) We computed two regression analyses between the scores obtained by subjects in the MRT and the degree of CBF increases. All results for the Z maps were thresholded at $p < .001$ (uncorrected for multiple comparisons) and are displayed in Table 5. Regarding the object imagery tasks,

TABLE 5

Peak coordinates of the significant positive regression between the MRT scores and blood flow values during object and spatial imagery tasks as compared to baseline conditions ($p < .001$, uncorrected for multiple comparisons)

Anatomical location of max. voxel activation	Coordinates			Z-score	$r_{(12)}$
	x	y	z		
Object MRT positive					
L. olfactory gyrus	−4	12	−16	4.5	0.923
L. putamen	−14	14	−10	3.5	0.825
R. thalamus	16	−18	14	3.9	0.875
L. inferior parietal gyrus/angular gyrus	−46	−58	42	4.3	0.906
L. cuneus/calcarine fissure	−4	−94	16	3.7	0.857
Spatial MRT positive					
R. cerebellum VIII	20	−72	−48	4.4	0.540
R. cerebellum VIII	34	−60	−54	3.3	0.419
R. cerebellum Crus II	42	−62	−48	3.3	0.417
L. cerebellum Crus I	−42	−64	−38	4.1	0.504
L. cerebellum Crus I	−28	−66	−32	3.2	0.410
R. cerebellum VIII	32	−36	−52	4.0	0.498
L. cerebellum VI	22	−66	−18	3.6	0.453
R. thalamus	12	−12	2	3.6	0.455
L. precuneus	2	−62	32	3.8	0.481
R. supramarginal gyrus	62	−46	34	3.8	0.470
R. angular gyrus	62	−56	36	3.3	0.419
R. anterior insula	46	18	−6	3.7	0.460
R. anterior insula	42	16	−14	3.5	0.445
R. inferior frontal sulcus	42	12	30	3.8	0.479
L. inferior frontal sulcus	−48	22	28	3.2	0.412
L. superior temporal gyrus	−58	−26	16	3.5	0.440
R. superior temporal gyrus	52	−30	18	3.2	0.409

The anatomical localisation of the maximum Z-scores of these regions is given on the basis of the MNI template, using their stereotactic coordinates in mm (R: right; L: left).

Figure 2 (opposite). (A) Plots show the activation of calcarine cortex during object imagery tasks (pink) and deactivation of calcarine cortex during spatial imagery tasks (blue) (x = −2, y = −102, z = 10 and x = 8, y = −88, z = 12). (B) Sagittal slice showing significant positive regression, in the calcarine cortex, between blood flow values during object imagery as compared to baseline and the MRT scores ($p < .001$). (C) 3-D rendering of the statistical map showing significant positive regressions between MRT scores and blood flow values in spatial imagery tasks as compared to baseline ($p < .001$). Plots show the positive regression between imagery conditions and MRT scores in areas indicated by arrows (see Table 5).

A

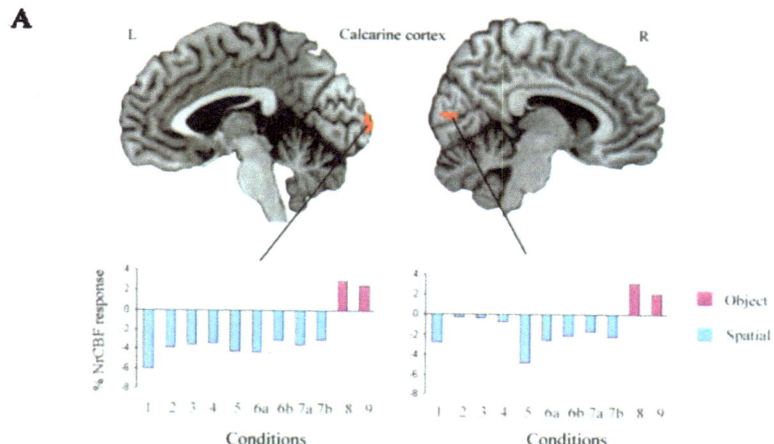

B

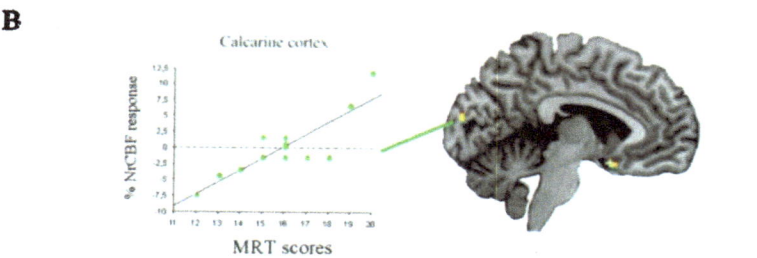

C

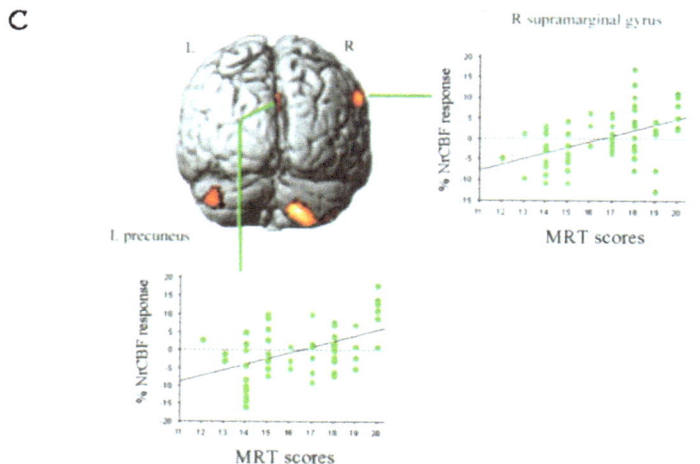

we found that CBF increases were positively correlated with the MRT scores in the left angular gyrus and in the dorsal bank of the left calcarine fissure.

Positive correlations in the spatial imagery tasks were found between MRT scores and activation in the cerebellar cortex bilaterally, the left inferior parietal lobe including the precuneus, the angular gyrus and the supramarginal gyrus, the right anterior insula, the bilateral inferior frontal sulcus and the left and right superior temporal gyrus.

DISCUSSION

The purpose of the present study was to assess the neural bases of two different types of mental imagery tasks as revealed by a multistudy of a large set of PET scans. We focused on three sets of results. The first set reflected the neural substrate common to both spatial and object imagery tasks, as revealed by a conjunction analysis. The second set of results compared each type of mental imagery (spatial and object), providing a direct measure of the effects of the tasks on brain areas involved in visual mental imagery. The third set of results explored the relationships between CBF increases and the individual ability of the subjects for mental imagery.

Common activations for object and spatial imagery conditions

Ventral and dorsal visual pathways.   The first finding, in agreement with numerous previous reports, was that object and spatial imagery activated both ventral and dorsal visual pathways (Mellet et al., 1998). However, our results did not contradict the classical functional dichotomy between the ''what'' and ''where'' pathways putatively used in mental imagery. Rather, they indicated that even when the tasks are designed specifically to draw on spatial processing, they require some object processing and vice versa. The involvement of both dorsal and ventral pathways has been previously reported in spatial mental imagery (Larsen, Bundesen, Kyllingsbaek, Paulson, & Law, 2000; Roland & Gulyas, 1995) and also in object mental imagery tasks (Ishai et al., 2000; Kosslyn et al., 1997; Lambert et al., 2002). As emphasised by Kosslyn, this finding underlines that pure forms of imagery are rare (Kosslyn et al., 1997). For example, in the present analysis, the spatial imagery task of Condition 2 required the subjects to generate images of 3-D objects based on spatial instructions. Moreover, in the object imagery condition, 9, the subjects were to adjust and to add details to their mental image according to the verbal description they heard. These ''online'' modifications are likely to rely in part on spatial processing.

Frontal lobe.   The activations detected in the frontal lobe overlapped clearly those observed in tasks that involve working memory (Haxby, Petit, Ungerleider, & Courtney, 2000; for a review, see Owen, 2000) and retrieval from episodic memory (see Nyberg, 1998, for review; Buckner & Wheeler, 2001). These common activations reflect the fact that mental imagery, working memory and retrieval from episodic memory share common cognitive processes—and also underscore the fact that these three cognitive functions are difficult to disentangle. Baddeley has formalised the relationships between working and episodic memory in a revised version of his model, which now includes an episodic buffer (Baddeley, 2000). The generation of mental images commonly relies on the reactivation of representation stored in episodic memory, a process equivalent to retrieval (Buckner & Wheeler, 2001). Along the same lines, mental image maintenance appears very close, if not identical, to visuospatial working memory (Kosslyn, 1994). Indeed, the phenomenal experience of mental imagery could be seen as the result of an interaction between the retrieval of visual representations from episodic memory and the maintenance and transformation properties of working memory and may be revealed, in part, by the present frontal activation.

In addition to the frontal involvement, some other activations supported the participation of a memory network. These activations occurred in the anterior insular cortex, which has been shown to belong to an episodic memory network (Donaldson, Petersen, Ollinger, & Buckner, 2001). Moreover, reciprocal connections between the frontal lobe and the insular cortex have been well documented (Augustine, 1996). The anterior cingulate cortex also exhibited activation common to both spatial and object imagery tasks. This area has been reported as being activated in very different demanding cognitive tasks such as working memory and episodic retrieval (Cabeza & Nyberg, 2000; Duncan & Owen, 2000), and reflects a key role in evaluative processes (MacDonald, Cohen, Stenger, & Carter, 2000). It is likely that all the imagery tasks included in the present review required such processes. As a matter of fact, subjects performed the tasks in total darkness and were instructed to generate and maintain highly vivid and accurate mental images that rely on episodic and working memory.

The conscious experience of imagery probably does not arise from activation in frontal, insular, or cingulate cortex activity, but rather is likely to arise from the interaction of the frontal and anterior insular cortex (for the retrieval activity proper) with the associative visual areas belonging to the ventral pathway. This view is in agreement with Fuster's (1998) proposal that memory requires an interaction between the anterior cortex for executive memory and the posterior cortex for perceptual memory.

Differences between object and spatial imagery conditions

Early visual cortex.   Our findings of an activation of the early visual cortex, which is specific to object imagery tasks, may be controversial. It has been shown, in the model originally proposed by Kosslyn, that the visual buffer is used to reconstruct the local geometry of the surface of visualised objects or scenes (Kosslyn, 1994) and would thus be implemented within the early visual cortex. However, this activation together with the deactivation observed in spatial imagery tasks that we have already reported (Mazard et al., 2002; Mellet et al., 2000b), questions the exact role of the visual buffer. Kosslyn has recently suggested that mental images relying on spatial relations do not involve the visual buffer and that inspecting details of a mental image would be critical for the involvement of primary visual cortex (Kosslyn & Thompson, 2003). The present findings are thus compatible with this adaptation of the model. Note, however, that, as mentioned above, the mental images generated by the subjects during the spatial imagery tasks were not devoid of object features. Indeed the activation of the ventral pathway was observed in both types of imagery. Nevertheless, it is likely that successfully performing the tasks did not require an accurate evocation of shapes, colours, and textures incorporated in the mental image, a critical function of the visual buffer (Kosslyn et al., 2001; Thompson et al., 2001). Our results thus confirm that the type of imagery is a crucial feature for explaining the discrepancies among studies as well as the fact that most of the studies that reported activation in the early visual cortex dealt with object mental imagery (Bookheimer, Zeffiro, Blaxton, Gaillard, Malow, & Theodore, 1998; Klein, Paradis, Poline, Kosslyn, & Le Bihan, 2000; Kosslyn, Thompson, Kim, & Alpert, 1995; Kosslyn, Thompson, Kim, Rauch, & Alpert, 1996; Lambert et al., 2002).

Parietal cortex. Although present in both types of imagery tasks, the bilateral intraparietal sulcus was more activated in spatial imagery than in object imagery. The parietal activation reported here was located in the medial part of the intraparietal sulcus, including the precuneus. This localisa-tion was in agreement with results recently reported that documented the fact that visuospatial tasks, such as attentional shifts and visually guided saccades, activated the medial part of the intraparietal sulcus (Simon, Mangin, Cohen, Le Bihan, & Dehaene, 2002). The present parietal activation thus suggests that spatial attention processes played a particularly important role in spatial imagery tasks.

Frontal cortex. Very few significant differences were detected in the frontal lobes in the comparison between the two types of tasks, suggesting that the type of images processed does not affect frontal activations. Frontal activation may mainly reflect processes common to both categories of tasks. Retrieval from episodic memory and maintenance in working memory are the most obvious such processes. The only major difference revealed that a region located at the intersection of the left precentral sulcus and the superior frontal sulcus was more activated in spatial imagery than in object imagery tasks. Activation of this region has been reported in various spatial working memory tasks (Courtney, Petit, Maisog, Ungerleider, & Haxby, 1998; Jonides, Smith, Koeppe, Awh,

Minoshima, & Mintun, 1993; Smith, Jonides, Koeppe, Awh, Schumacher, & Minoshima, 1995). Its activation during spatial imagery tasks is likely to reflect the large amount of spatial transformations required.

Left inferior temporal/fusiform cortex.   We observed an activation of the left inferior temporal cortex specific to the object imagery tasks. This large activation spread from the left occipitotemporal sulcus to the left parahippocampal cortex and the left hippocampus. Using direct single neuron recordings in humans, a recent study has demonstrated that the hippocampus and the entorhinal cortex are involved in mental image generation of objects and faces (Kreiman, Koch, & Fried, 2000). Moreover, it has been suggested that this anterior part of the ventral visual pathway is engaged in multimodal integration, particularly between language and visual perception (Büchel, Price, & Friston, 1998; Papathanassiou, Etard, Mellet, Zago, Mazoyer, & Tzourio-Mazoyer, 2000; Price, 2000). It has been claimed that activations in this region raise "the intriguing possibility that semantic or conceptual representations of words may also be accessed directly within the ventral pathway" (Nobre, Allison, & McCarthy, 1994, p. 262). Our findings are compatible with this suggestion. In fact, in the two studies dealing with object imagery included in the present analysis, the image generation process was driven by linguistic stimuli (as reflected by the primary and secondary auditory cortex activation): single words in Study 8 and descriptive sentences in Study 9.

In the present analysis, a leftward lateralisation was evident in the ventral pathway activation only when imagery of concrete items (object imagery) was compared to spatial imagery. This observation sheds light on the hemispheric lateralisation of mental imagery, an issue that remains unclear. It suggests that a strong component of object imagery is a prerequisite for a leftward lateralisation. Moreover, it supports a previous proposition that the left-lateralised ventral activation reflects the integration process between language and the retrieval processes required for imagery of concrete items (Mellet et al., 1998; Wise et al., 2000).

Individual variability

All subjects included in the present analysis were selected on the basis of their high scores obtained in the MRT. Although restricted to a sample of subjects who scored from 12 to 20 on the MRT (thus categorised as "high visuospatial imagers"), the correlations between the MRT scores and the amount of CBF increase during various imagery tasks begin to address the issue of the neural correlates of individual variability in visual imagery.

A first result showed that the better the subjects performed on the MRT, the higher their activation in the primary visual cortex during object imagery tasks. Negative correlations between reaction time and activation have been previously reported (Klein et al., 2000; Kosslyn et al., 1996), which indicated that the fastest responses were associated with a more pronounced activation in the primary visual cortex. Taken together, these results emphasise that early visual cortex is affected by individual variability of imagery skills, a fact that should be considered when trying to explain discrepancies observed between studies.

Turning now to the spatial imagery tasks, significant positive correlations were evident in the inferior parietal cortex, anterior insular cortex, and precuneus. Activation in this set of cerebral regions was also evident in the conjunction analysis that included both the spatial and object imagery conditions. These areas were thought to be involved in the memory component of the imagery tasks. The present result suggests that this network is involved during both object and spatial imagery conditions and its activation varies according to one's individual imagery abilities.

Finally, CBF increases were positively correlated with imagery ability in the left parietal lobe in object imagery tasks whereas this correlation was with the right parietal lobe in the spatial imagery tasks. This observation may indicate that "high imagers" recruit substantially more effective brain regions than "lower performers" while performing imagery tasks. Consistent with this possibility, it has been suggested that the left parietal cortex is involved in image generation whereas the right parietal cortex is preferentially engaged in mental image manipulation that often characterises spatial imagery (Formisano et al., 2002).

CONCLUSIONS

We took advantage of a PET multistudy database of 54 subjects. The common pattern of activation of object and spatial imagery strongly implicates both the ventral and dorsal routes, regardless of the nature of the task. There is, however, variation in the level of activity in different tasks. Object imagery relied specifically on the anterior part of the ventral route, which may partly reflect the interaction between language and imagery. On the other hand, the dorsal route seemed to be more activated by the spatial than by the object imagery tasks, in agreement with its preferential role in the processing of spatial information. Finally, our study provides new insights regarding the debate about the involvement of the early visual cortex in mental imagery. First, it offers evidence that the early visual cortex (although not necessary for all types of imagery) may play a role in the imagery of figurative attributes. Secondly, the activity of the early visual cortex during the object imagery tasks varied among subjects. This finding provides evidence of the functional interindividual variability within the early visual cortex during object imagery. This functional variability should be taken into account in order to explain the divergent results found in previous studies.

PrEview proof published online May 2004

REFERENCES

Augustine, J. R. (1996). Circuitry and functional aspects of the insular lobe in primates including humans. *Brain Research Reviews, 22,* 229–244.

Baddeley, A. (2000). The episodic buffer: A new component of working memory? *Trends in Cognitive Sciences, 4,* 417–423.

Bookheimer, S. Y., Zeffiro, T. A., Blaxton, T. A., Gaillard, W. D., Malow, B., & Theodore, W. H. (1998). Regional cerebral blood flow during auditory responsive naming: Evidence for cross-modality neural activation. *Neuroreport, 9,* 2409–2413.

Büchel, C., Price, C., & Friston, K. (1998). A multimodal language region in the ventral visual pathway. *Nature, 394,* 274–277.

Buckner, R. L., & Wheeler, M. E. (2001). The cognitive neuroscience of remembering. *Nature Reviews Neuroscience, 2,* 624–634.

Cabeza, R., & Nyberg, L. (2000). Imaging cognition II: An empirical review of 275 PET and fMRI studies. *Journal of Cognitive Neuroscience, 12,* 1–47.

Courtney, S. M., Petit, L., Maisog, J. M., Ungerleider, L. G., & Haxby, J. V. (1998). An area specialized for spatial working memory in human frontal cortex. *Science, 279,* 1347–1351.

Donaldson, D. I., Petersen, S. E., Ollinger, J. M., & Buckner, R. L. (2001). Dissociating state and item components of recognition memory using fMRI. *NeuroImage, 13,* 129–142.

Duncan, J., & Owen, A. M. (2000). Common regions of the human frontal lobe recruited by diverse cognitive demands. *Trends in Neurosciences, 23,* 475–483.

Farah, M. J. (1984). The neurological basis of mental imagery: A componential analysis. *Cognition, 18,* 245–272.

Formisano, E., Linden, D. E., Di Salle, F., Trojano, L., Esposito, F., Sack, A. T., Grossi, D., Zanella, F. E., & Goebel, R. (2002). Tracking the mind's image in the brain I. Time-resolved fMRI during visuospatial mental imagery. *Neuron, 35,* 185–194.

Friston, K., Holmes, A., Poline, J.-B., Frith, C. D., & Frackowiak, R. S. J. (1995). Statistical parametric maps in functional imaging: A general linear approach. *Human Brain Mapping, 2,* 189–210.

Friston, K. J., Holmes, A. P., Price, C. J., Büchel, C., & Worsley, K. J. (1999). Multisubject fMRI studies and conjunction analyses. *NeuroImage, 10,* 385–396.

Fuster, J. M. (1998). Linkage at the top. *Neuron, 21,* 1223–1224.

Ghaëm, O., Mellet, E., Crivello, F., Tzourio, N., Mazoyer, B., Berthoz, A., & Denis, M. (1997). Mental navigation along memorized routes activates the hippocampus, precuneus, and insula. *Neuroreport, 8,* 739–744.

Gusnard, D. A., & Raichle, M. E. (2001). Searching for a baseline: Functional imaging and the resting human brain. *Nature Reviews Neuroscience, 2,* 685–694.

Haxby, J. V., Petit, L., Ungerleider, L. G., & Courtney, S. M. (2000). Distinguishing the functional roles of multiple regions in distributed neural systems for visual working memory. *NeuroImage, 11,* 145–156.

Ishai, A., Ungerleider, L. G., & Haxby, J. V. (2000). Distributed neural systems for the generation of visual images. *Neuron, 28,* 979–990.

Jonides, J., Smith, E. E., Koeppe, R. A., Awh, E., Minoshima, S., & Mintun, M. A. (1993). Spatial working memory in humans as revealed by PET. *Nature, 363,* 623–625.

Klein, I., Paradis, A. L., Poline, J. B., Kosslyn, S. M., & Le Bihan, D. (2000). Transient activity in the human calcarine cortex during visual–mental imagery: An event-related fMRI study. *Journal of Cognitive Neuroscience, 12*(Suppl. 2), 15–23.

Kosslyn, S. M. (1987). Seeing and imagining in the cerebral hemispheres: A computational approach. *Psychological Review, 94,* 148–175.

Kosslyn, S. M. (1994). *Image and brain: The resolution of the imagery debate.* Cambridge, MA: MIT Press.

Kosslyn, S. M., Alpert, N. M., Thompson, W. L., Maljkovic, V., Weise, S. B., Chabris, C. F., Hamilton, S. E., Rauch, S. L., & Buonanno, F. S. (1993). Visual mental imagery activates topographically organised visual cortex: PET investigations. *Journal of Cognitive Neuroscience, 5*, 263–287.

Kosslyn, S. M., Ganis, G., & Thompson, W. L. (2001). Neural foundations of imagery. *Nature Reviews Neuroscience, 2*, 635–642.

Kosslyn, S. M., & Ochsner, K. N. (1994). In search of occipital activation during visual mental imagery. *Trends in Neurosciences, 17*, 290–292.

Kosslyn, S. M., & Thompson, W. L. (2003). When is early visual cortex activated during visual mental imagery? Theory and meta-analysis. *Psychological Bulletin, 129*, 723–746.

Kosslyn, S. M., Thompson, W. L., & Alpert, N. M. (1997). Neural systems shared by visual imagery and visual perception: A positron emission tomography study. *NeuroImage, 6*, 320–334.

Kosslyn, S. M., Thompson, W. L., Kim, I. J., & Alpert, N. M. (1995). Topographical representations of mental images in primary visual cortex. *Nature, 378*, 496–498.

Kosslyn, S. M., Thompson, W. L., Kim, I. J., Rauch, S. L., & Alpert, N. M. (1996). Individual differences in cerebral blood flow in area 17 predict the time to evaluate visualized letters. *Journal of Cognitive Neuroscience, 8*, 78–82.

Kreiman, G., Koch, C., & Fried, I. (2000). Imagery neurons in the human brain. *Nature, 408*, 357–361.

Lambert, S., Sampaio, E., Scheiber, C., & Mauss, Y. (2002). Neural substrates of animal mental imagery: Calcarine sulcus and dorsal pathway involvement—an fMRI study. *Brain Research, 924*, 176–183.

Larsen, A., Bundesen, C., Kyllingsbaek, S., Paulson, O. B., & Law, I. (2000). Brain activation during mental transformation of size. *Journal of Cognitive Neuroscience, 12*, 763–774.

MacDonald, A. W., III, Cohen, J. D., Stenger, V. A., & Carter, C. S. (2000). Dissociating the role of the dorsolateral prefrontal and anterior cingulate cortex in cognitive control. *Science, 288*, 1835–1838.

Mazard, A., Mazoyer, B., Etard, O., Tzourio-Mazoyer, N., Kosslyn, S. M., & Mellet, E. (2002). Impact of fMRI acoustic noise on the functional anatomy of visual mental imagery. *Journal of Cognitive Neuroscience, 14*, 172–186.

Mazoyer, B., Zago, L., Mellet, E., Bricogne, S., Etard, O., Houde, O., Crivello, F., Joliot, M., Petit, L., & Tzourio-Mazoyer, N. (2001). Cortical networks for working memory and executive functions sustain the conscious resting state in man. *Brain Research Bulletin, 54*, 287–298.

Mellet, E., Bricogne, S., Crivello, F., Mazoyer, B., Denis, M., & Tzourio-Mazoyer, N. (2002). Neural basis of mental scanning of a topographic representation built from a text. *Cerebral Cortex, 12*, 1322–1330.

Mellet, E., Bricogne, S., Tzourio-Mazoyer, N., Ghaëm, O., Petit, L., Zago, L., Etard, O., Berthoz, A., Mazoyer, B., & Denis, M. (2000a). Neural correlates of topographic mental exploration: The impact of route versus survey perspective learning. *NeuroImage, 12*, 588–600.

Mellet, E., Petit, L., Mazoyer, B., Denis, M., & Tzourio, N. (1998). Reopening the mental imagery debate: Lessons from functional anatomy. *NeuroImage, 8*, 129–139.

Mellet, E., Tzourio-Mazoyer, N., Bricogne, S., Mazoyer, B., Kosslyn, S. M., & Denis, M. (2000b). Functional anatomy of high-resolution visual mental imagery. *Journal of Cognitive Neuroscience, 12*, 98–109.

Mellet, E., Tzourio, N., Crivello, F., Joliot, M., Denis, M., & Mazoyer, B. (1996). Functional anatomy of spatial mental imagery generated from verbal instructions. *Journal of Neuroscience, 16*, 6504–6512.

Mellet, E., Tzourio, N., Denis, M., & Mazoyer, B. (1995). A positron emission tomography study of visual and mental spatial exploration. *Journal of Cognitive Neuroscience, 7*, 433–445.

Mellet, E., Tzourio, N., Denis, M., & Mazoyer, B. (1998). Cortical anatomy of mental imagery of concrete nouns based on their dictionary definition. *Neuroreport, 9*, 803–808.

Nobre, A. C., Allison, T., & McCarthy, G. (1994). Word recognition in the human inferior temporal lobe. *Nature, 372*, 260–263.

Nyberg, L. (1998). Mapping episodic memory. *Behavioural Brain Research, 90*, 107–114.

Oldfield, R. C. (1971). The assessment and analysis of handedness: The Edinburgh inventory. *Neuropsychologia, 9*, 97–113.

Owen, A. M. (2000). The role of the lateral frontal cortex in mnemonic processing: The contribution of functional neuroimaging. *Experimental Brain Research, 133*, 33–43.

Papathanassiou, D., Etard, O., Mellet, E., Zago, L., Mazoyer, B., & Tzourio-Mazoyer, N. (2000). A common language network for comprehension and production: A contribution to the definition of language epicenters with PET. *NeuroImage, 11*, 347–357.

Price, C. J. (2000). The anatomy of language: Contributions from functional neuroimaging. *Journal of Anatomy, 197*(Pt. 3), 335–359.

Price, C. J., & Friston, K. J. (1997). Cognitive conjunction: A new approach to brain activation experiments. *NeuroImage, 5*, 261–270.

Roland, P. E., & Gulyas, B. (1994). Visual imagery and visual representation. *Trends in Neurosciences, 17*, 281–287.

Roland, P. E., & Gulyas, B. (1995). Visual memory, visual imagery, and visual recognition of large field patterns by the human brain: Functional anatomy by positron emission tomography. *Cerebral Cortex, 5*, 79–93.

Sakai, K., & Miyashita, Y. (1994). Visual imagery: An interaction between memory retrieval and focal attention. *Trends in Neurosciences, 17*, 287–289.

Shepard, R. N., & Metzler, J. (1971). Mental rotation of three-dimensional objects. *Science, 171*, 701–703.

Simon, O., Mangin, J. F., Cohen, L., Le Bihan, D., & Dehaene, S. (2002). Topographical layout of hand, eye, calculation, and language-related areas in the human parietal lobe. *Neuron, 33*, 475–487.

Smith, E. E., Jonides, J., Koeppe, R. A., Awh, E., Schumacher, E. H., & Minoshima, S. (1995). Spatial versus object working memory: PET investigations. *Journal of Cognitive Neuroscience, 7*, 337–356.

Taylor, H. A., & Tversky, B. (1992). Spatial mental models derived from survey and route description descriptions. *Journal of Memory and Language, 31*, 261–292.

Thompson, W. L., Kosslyn, S. M., Sukel, K. E., & Alpert, N. M. (2001). Mental imagery of high- and low-resolution gratings activates area 17. *NeuroImage, 14*, 454–464.

Tzourio-Mazoyer, N., Landeau, B., Papathanassiou, D., Crivello, F., Etard, O., Delcroix, N., Mazoyer, B., & Joliot, M. (2002). Automated anatomical labeling of activations in SPM using a macroscopic anatomical parcellation of the MNI MRI single-subject brain. *NeuroImage, 15*, 273–289.

Vandenberg, S. G., & Kuse, A. R. (1978). Mental rotations, a group test of three-dimensional spatial visualization. *Perceptual and Motor Skills, 47*, 599–604.

Wise, R. J., Howard, D., Mummery, C. J., Fletcher, P., Leff, A., Büchel, C., & Scott, S. K. (2000). Noun imageability and the temporal lobes. *Neuropsychologia, 38*, 985–994.

Woods, R. P., Grafton, S. T., Holmes, C. J., Cherry, S. R., & Mazziotta, J. C. (1998). Automated image registration: I. General methods and intrasubject, intramodality validation. *Journal of Computer Assisted Tomography, 22*, 139–152.

EUROPEAN JOURNAL OF COGNITIVE PSYCHOLOGY, 2004, *16* (5), 696–716

Brain rCBF and performance in visual imagery tasks: Common and distinct processes

Stephen M. Kosslyn

Department of Psychology, Harvard University, Cambridge, and Department of Neurology, Massachusetts General Hospital, Boston, MA, USA

William L. Thompson and Jennifer M. Shephard

Department of Psychology, Harvard University, Cambridge, MA, USA

Giorgio Ganis

Department of Psychology, Harvard University, Cambridge, and Department of Radiology, Massachusetts General Hospital, Boston, MA, USA

Deborah Bell

Department of Psychology, Harvard University, Cambridge, MA, USA

Judith Danovitch

Department of Psychology, Yale University, New Haven, CT, USA

Leah A. Wittenberg

University of British Columbia Medical School, Vancouver, BC, Canada

Nathaniel M. Alpert

Department of Radiology, Massachusetts General Hospital, Boston, MA, USA

The present study was designed to discover whether variations in normalised regional cerebral blood flow (rCBF) in different brain areas predict variations in performance of different imagery tasks. Positron emission tomography (PET) was used to assess brain activity as 16 participants performed four imagery tasks. These tasks were designed so that performance was particularly sensitive to the participant's ability to form images with high resolution, to generate images from distinct segments, to parse imaged forms into parts while inspecting them, or to transform (rotate) images. Response times and error rates were recorded. Multiple regression

Correspondence should be addressed to S. M. Kosslyn, Harvard Univ. Psychology Dept, 832 William James Hall, 33 Kirkland Street, Cambridge, MA 02138, USA. Email: smk@wjh.harvard.edu

This research was supported by AFOSR Grant F49620 98-1-0334; DOD Contract NMA201-01-C-0032; NSF Grant REC-0106760; and NIH grant 5 R01 MH60734.

http://www.tandf.co.uk/journals/pp/09541446.html   DOI: 10.1080/09541440340000475

analyses revealed that variations in most brain areas predicted variations in performance of only one task, thus demonstrating that the four tasks tap largely independent imagery processes. However, we also found that some underlying processes were recruited by more than one task, particularly those implemented in the occipito-parietal sulcus, the medial frontal cortex, and Area 18.

One of the major virtues of neuroimaging is that it can illuminate the structure of neural information processing systems. Many cognitive faculties—such as language, perception, and imagery—have been shown not to be unitary, but rather to be accomplished by a host of processes working in concert (e.g., Kandel & Squire, 2000; Kosslyn, Thompson, & Alpert, 1997; Mellet, Petit, Mazoyer, Denis, & Tzourio, 1998; Smith & Jonides, 1997). Neuroimaging is a powerful method for discovering whether distinct processes carry out different tasks (Kosslyn, 1999). In some cases, neuroimaging has revealed that tasks that appear very different are in fact accomplished by many of the same underlying processes. For example, the tasks of visualising upper-case letters and naming pictured objects seen from unusual viewpoints activate approximately two-thirds of the same brain areas (Kosslyn et al., 1997).

Such findings not only underscore the commonalities among tasks, but also reveal ways in which they differ. Thus, in the case of imagery and perception, we can begin to understand why brain damage often affects the two faculties together—but sometimes spares one or the other (Behrmann, Moscovitch, & Winocur, 1994; Farah, 1984). All else being equal, if about two-thirds of the same areas are shared, we would expect brain damage to disrupt both functions together more often than one but not the other—and many examples in the clinical literature seem to suggest that this is the case (Bisiach & Luzatti, 1978; Farah, 1984, 2000).

Neuroimaging is typically used to study the structure of neural information processing by relying on, essentially, a subtractive logic. Researchers ask participants to take part in two (or more) tasks, and for each comparison one task is treated as the experimental task and another as the baseline. Researchers then compare the pattern of regional cerebral blood flow (rCBF) or relative activation in the two tasks. For example, one might conduct an imagery task and compare the results from it to those from a resting baseline or from a simple eye fixation task. The goal is to isolate the neural bases of a subset of the processes used in the experimental task by removing the contribution of processes used in the other task. However, life is not so simple: The problem is that we don't know which processes are involved in either task—the experimental or baseline. Although the baseline task typically seems simpler than the experimental task, there is no guarantee that it in fact relies on a proper subset of the processes used in the experimental task. Thus, it is not clear what is being removed by the subtraction. This problem is related to the classic ''fallacy of pure insertion'', where researchers realised that different operations could be performed when tasks were simplified (see Boring, 1950, pp. 148–149; Külpe, 1895, pp. 406–422; Luce, 1986, pp. 212–217; Woodworth, 1938, pp. 309–310).

The subtractive neuroimaging method is designed to answer a specific question, namely "What set of brain areas is active while one performs a specific task?" But this is not the only question one can address with neuroimaging. In addition, one can ask: "Which set of brain areas underlies *variations in performance* of a specific task?" Rather than seek to discover the entire set of areas that is active during a task, this second question focuses only on a subset; we now ask which areas, when they are more strongly activated, are associated with better or worse performance in a particular task? Rather than use a subtractive logic, this question is best addressed with a multiple regression logic.

To our knowledge, the first neuroimaging study of imagery to use the regression approach was reported by Kosslyn, Thompson, Kim, Rauch, and Alpert (1996). They scanned the brains of 16 participants, using positron emission tomography (PET), while the participants visualised upper-case letters and then decided whether each had specific properties (such as any curved lines). Response times (RTs) and error rates (ERs) were collected during scanning. These behavioural dependent measures later were regressed onto measures of rCBF in a set of regions of interest (ROIs) recorded during the task. Multiple regression analysis revealed that rCBF in three brain areas accounted for approximately 88% of the variance in RTs. However, Kosslyn et al. used only one task; it is possible that any imagery task would have produced the same results, or that only that specific task would produce those results.

In the present study, we use the regression logic to ask whether different processes regulate performance in different visual imagery tasks. We designed four tasks with an eye towards tapping a subset of distinct processes in each. Our logic relied on the idea that processes can be divided into two classes (Kosslyn & Plomin, 2001). Consider the following analogy: When typing, variations in the strength of fingers are not relevant; provided one has a well-designed keyboard, one can type effectively if one has a minimal level of finger strength—anything more than that is irrelevant. In contrast, one's ability to plan ahead will affect typing speed, as will how quickly one can execute motor commands. Thus, one class of processes is "minimally sufficient": given that one can perform them at all, additional facility with those processes will not improve performance on that task. In contrast, another class of processes is "rate limiting": improved performance of those processes leads to improved performance of the task. Note that the relation of the processes to the task is crucial: the same process can be minimally sufficient for one task and rate limiting for another. By analogy, in direct contradistinction to typing, the ease of opening the lid of a jar does vary depending on finger strength, but not on the ease of planning ahead or speed in motor commands.

Our goal was to design visual imagery tasks that incorporated different rate-limiting processes; we designed the tasks so that they drew more or less heavily on these processes. The specific processes of interest were inspired by the results of a study of individual differences in imagery (Kosslyn, Brunn, Cave, & Wallach, 1984). This study led us to focus on four classes of processes, as follows: *image resolution*, which is the ability to represent and interpret patterns with high resolution; *image generation*, which is the ability to compose patterns in mental images based on stored information; *image inspection*, which is the ability to interpret patterns in images; and *image transformation*, which is the ability to alter patterns in images, such as in mental rotation. Mast and Kosslyn (2002) used performance on these tasks to predict performance on an entirely different task; specifically, as expected, only performance on the image transformation task predicted which participants could mentally rotate an ambiguous figure of a face and "see" its alternative interpretation. Thus, the tasks have some measure of validity, and it makes sense to investigate the neural processes they recruit.

Participants performed all four tasks as their brains were scanned using PET. We chose to use PET in this study for two main reasons: First, rCBF measures may be more closely coupled with neural activation than the blood oxygenation level dependent (BOLD) measures obtained with functional magnetic resonance imaging (fMRI), and thus be less sensitive to between-participant noise (cf. Aguirre, Detre, Zarahn, & Alsop, 2002). Second, we wanted to sample the entire brain, which is still a challenge with fMRI perfusion methods (e.g., Detre & Wang, 2002).

We collected RTs and ERs while the participants performed each task. Later, we performed a two-stage analysis. First, we analysed covariance of these behavioural measures with normalised rCBF, which allowed us to identify a set of brain regions. We partialled out the effects of participants' scores on the Advanced Progressive Matrices Test (Raven, Raven, & Court, 1998). Regions of interest were traced around the locus of maximal rCBF for each identified area and an rCBF value was then extracted for each area for each of the replicates of each task. We obtained values for all tasks in all areas that were identified in any of the tasks. Thus, eight values were obtained for each region. Second, we then performed a forward stepwise multiple regression analysis to identify brain regions that contributed unique variance in accounting for variations in behavioural performance. The regression analyses were performed separately for the two replicates, given the results of the behavioural data and the possible effects of practice. In addition, separate regression analyses were performed with RT and with ER as the dependent measure. Thus, each of the initially identified regions was entered into four regression analyses for each task. We asked whether variations in rCBF of different brain areas predicted performance in the different tasks.

We expected performance in the resolution task to depend on the efficacy of representing fine spatial variations in topographically organised cortex, Areas 17 or 18; we expected performance in the image generation task to rely largely on dorsolateral prefrontal areas, along with Area 19, posterior parietal, and inferior temporal areas (see Kosslyn et al., 1997); we expected performance in the inspection task to rely on frontal and inferior frontal areas, as well as topographically organised cortex; and we expected performance in the rotation task to rely primarily on posterior parietal cortex (e.g., Cohen et al., 1996). However, all of these predictions are based on studies that used the subtractive logic. It really is an open question which processes are rate limiting and which are minimally sufficient. The present study represents a first effort to begin exploring this uncharted territory.

METHOD

Participants

Sixteen people (eight female, eight male, mean age 21 years, range 18–28 years) volunteered to participate in this study for pay. All participants provided informed consent and completed a health history questionnaire before they took part in this study. None of the participants reported health problems and all had normal or corrected-to-normal vision. The participants were undergraduate or graduate students (most from Harvard University) or professionals from the Boston area. No participant was aware of the purpose of this study until debriefing.

Materials

We used the Psyscope (Cohen, MacWhinney, Flatt, & Provost, 1993) program to present the four tasks while rCBF was recorded using PET. All tasks shared the same basic trial design: First, a circle appeared, which contained three radii that divided it into three equal-sized wedges. This "Mercedes symbol" was oriented in different ways in different stimuli. As illustrated in Figure 1, the boundary of the circle differed for the three wedges: For one wedge, the boundary was heavy black; for another, it was dashed; and for the third wedge, the boundary was a fine line. The participants always had to compare the portions of imaged characters that fell in the wedge bordered by the heavy black line with the portions that fell in the wedge bordered by the dashed line. For all four tasks, we included a total of 36 trials (18 unique trials were repeated in such a way that no one trial was repeated before all 18 had been seen). We used 21 alphanumeric characters for the imagery tasks; 18 were test items, which appeared between 4 and 28 times. In addition, stimuli were designed so that on half the trials in each task more of the cued character would be in the dashed-boundary wedge and on half the trials more of the character would be in the thick black-boundary wedge. The trials were arranged so that no more than three in succession had more of the character in the wedge with the same boundary. We prepared 16 practice trials, four for each task; these trials had the identical form as the test trials

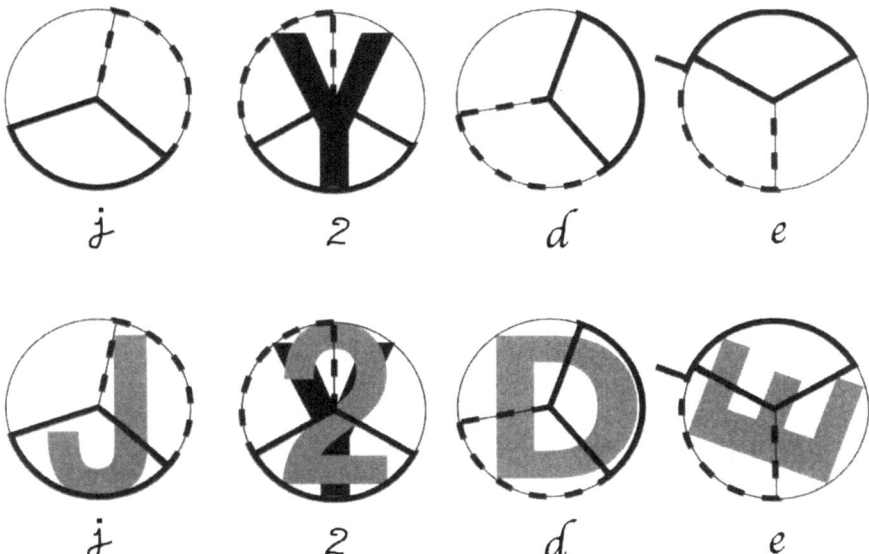

Figure 1. An illustration of sample stimuli for the resolution, generation, inspection, and transformation tasks, respectively. The top line of pictures depicts actual stimuli as presented to participants for each task; in the bottom line of pictures the grey character represents the image participants would need to form in order to make the judgement appropriate for each task (the answers are *bold, bold, dashed, dashed*, respectively). In all tasks except the inspection task, participants were asked to judge whether more of the total area of the imaged character (or imaged character plus character already present, in the case of the generation task) would appear within the bold section or the dashed section of the circle. For the inspection task, the participants were asked to judge whether more segments of the imaged character would appear in the bold or dashed section of the circle.

except that during practice there was feedback for accuracy. If the participant responded incorrectly, the computer would beep and would not advance to the next trial until the response was corrected. During the experimental trials, there was no such feedback.

The tasks were constructed after a lengthy period of pilot testing. We administered longer versions of these tasks iteratively to approximately 100 pilot participants, and used these results to select stimuli so that the final versions of the tasks had comparable overall mean ERs and RTs.

The materials used in each task were as follows: A study phase was presented at the beginning of the experiment, for which we prepared 17 simple upper case block letters and 4 numbers. Each character was presented in a circle, which measured approximately 4.5 cm in diameter.

Image resolution. For use in the test phase, we prepared trials with the following events: First, a circle appeared (at the same size as the circles that surrounded each character during the study phase) with a script character beneath it. The circle was divided into three equal wedges, and one wedge had a thick black boundary, one had a dashed boundary, and one had a thin boundary. We oriented the wedges so that if the cued block character were actually in the circle, very similar amounts of it would be in the wedge with the thick black boundary and the wedge with the dashed boundary. Thus, a high-resolution image would be necessary to perform the task well.

Image generation.   In this task, a mental image was to be superimposed over a character already printed within the circle, and the judgement made on the basis of the combined stimuli. Thus, the stimuli for this task were identical to those for the resolution task in all respects but two: First, we now actually included a character in the circle. The characters printed within the circles were drawn from the same set of 21 characters studied at the beginning of the experiment. On each trial, the character that was physically present within the circle and the one that was cued to be imaged were different, and thus the participants in all cases were required to form a novel image based on the combination. Second, we oriented the wedges so that one clearly would have more of the visible-character-plus-imaged-character if both were physically present; this meant that the discrimination itself was not difficult.

Image inspection.   The stimuli for this task were the same as those in the resolution task, with two changes: First, the wedges were not oriented so that more of a character's total area would be in one of the two key wedges, but rather so that more *segments* of a character would be in one of the wedges. A segment was defined as a stroke used to draw the character, for example, the upper-case letter A has three segments, the two diagonals and the horizontal. The stimuli were designed so that one wedge contained portions of more segments than the other. Second, we oriented the wedges so that the necessary discrimination was easy.

Image transformation.   Finally, the *transformation task* was essentially the same as the resolution task, but again with two changes: First, we now included a "tick mark" on the border of the circle. This tick was a cue that indicated how the participants should mentally rotate a visualised character. Second, again, the wedges were oriented so that one of the key wedges clearly had more of the character than the other, and thus the discrimination was not difficult once the character had been properly rotated.

Advanced Progressive Matrices Test.   We also administered Set I (practice) and Set II (untimed) of the Raven's Advanced Progressive Matrices (Raven et al., 1998). The test, which is a measure of general nonverbal intelligence (NVI), was completed approximately 1–2 weeks prior to the PET scanning session. Each participant received a score on the APM Set II (out of a possible total of

36, scores ranged from 23 to 36) and this score was considered a nuisance variable in the covariate analysis. Thus, we wished to discover areas in which variations in rCBF predicted performance in each of the tasks of interest, but independent of general nonverbal intelligence. We selected the Raven's test in part because, as noted by Duncan et al. (2000), it has often emerged from factor analyses as being highly correlated with general intelligence (''g''), and in part based on practical considerations—specifically, because it can be administered in a relatively short time (usually less than 1 hour), its instructions are easy to understand and apply to all trials, and participants may complete the test at their own rhythm and with relative independence. Although only some of the variance in NVI may be accounted for by an APM test score, it allowed us to remove at least some variability due to overall NVI; the results so construed were more likely to reflect accurately the processing in which we were most interested, namely the processes that subserved performance on our four tasks *per se*.

Procedure

We begin by summarising the behavioural procedure, and then review briefly the PET scanning procedure.

Behavioural procedure.   The participants first were settled into the bed of the scanner and fitted with a snug head and face mask, which prevented head movement (for details, see Kosslyn, Alpert, Thompson, Chabris, Rauch, & Anderson, 1994; Kosslyn, DiGirolamo, Thompson, & Alpert, 1998). They could clearly see a computer monitor that was positioned on a gantry; the monitor was approximately 55 cm from their eyes. At the outset of each task, the participants read instructions on the computer screen, and then were asked to paraphrase them aloud. Any misconceptions were corrected. They then received the stimuli for the study phase. We asked them to memorise the appearance of these characters in the following way: A character appeared on the screen within a circle for 5 s and then disappeared. The participants would then generate an image of the character in the empty circle. When they felt that they had formed an accurate image, they pressed a button and the character reappeared. They then compared their image to the character, so that they could correct any inaccuracies in their mental representation. This image formation-and-correction procedure was repeated before they proceeded to the next character.

Following this, we administered the instructions and four practice trials for the first task. Participants were to indicate their judgement by pressing one of two buttons (placed in their dominant hand); both the response and the RT were recorded by the computer. We interviewed the participants immediately after the practice trials to ensure that they understood the task; any misconceptions were corrected, and the participants were asked to paraphrase the instructions again. We asked the participants to make their judgements as quickly as possible, without sacrificing accuracy. PET scanning began only after the practice trials were complete and it was clear that the participant understood the task.

The participants received a block of trials for each of the four tasks before receiving a second set of blocks, in the same order. The same stimuli were used in both blocks for each of the four tasks, but the order of the stimuli was reversed in the second block. Thus, the participants received a total of eight blocks of trials. The order of the blocks was counterbalanced over the 16 participants, using a Latin square design, which ensured that each task appeared in each serial position equally often and each followed each other task equally often.

For the resolution task, we asked the participants to read the script cue, and then to visualise the corresponding block character in the circle, upright, and decide whether more of it would be in the wedge defined by the heavy black border or the wedge defined by the dashed line. Because the discrimination was difficult, the key rate-limiting steps in this task were the processes required to generate images with high resolution and to make fine discriminations while inspecting the image.

For the generation task, we asked the participants to meld the visualised character (cued by a script character beneath the stimulus) with the character that was printed within the circle. They were to decide which of the two key wedges would contain more of the combined characters, if both were actually present within the circle. Because the discrimination itself was relatively easy, the critical aspect of this task was the ability to compose shapes into a new whole.

For the inspection task, we asked the participants to decide which wedge would have more segments of the visualised character; each segment of a letter corresponds to a stroke typically made when drawing the block character. In the instructions we provided a diagram that illustrated how to decompose characters into segments and how to count the number of segments in a given wedge. Because the discrimination itself was easy, the critical aspects of this task were the abilities to parse the character into segments and compare the number of segments in each wedge.

For the transformation task, we asked the participants to read the cue, visualise the corresponding block character, and then mentally rotate the character until its top was directly under the tick mark. After rotating, the participants were to make the same discrimination required in the resolution task. However, in this case the discrimination was easy; the rate-limiting step in this task relied on processes that rotate the image.

In all cases, the trials were self-paced; the participants were permitted to respond to the trials at their own rate, and a participant's response triggered the appearance of the next trial. A fixation point appeared 50 ms after the start of each trial and remained on the screen for 500 ms; the stimulus appeared immediately following the fixation point. Response time measurement started with the appearance of the stimulus on the screen. We used a self-paced procedure for two reasons. First, we needed to maximise variability in performance across participants, and thus wanted to give participants the opportunity to perform more quickly—without being penalised by correspondingly longer delays between trials. Second, if we had chosen to present a fixed number of trials, the interstimulus interval (ISI) would need to be long enough to accommodate even relatively slow participants. This would have led the faster participants to spend proportionally more time during scanning waiting for the next stimulus, which would have affected rCBF unpredictably. A shorter ISI would have led to higher ER and speed–accuracy tradeoffs that would be difficult to interpret. Participants all spent an average of between 69 and 82 s of "integrated processing time" (total time actually performing the tasks) for each of the four tasks; the mean processing time was 75 s. The average number of trials per block completed by participants ranged from 12 to 29 (mean: 19).

PET procedure.   We have described the PET acquisition procedure in detail elsewhere (Kosslyn et al., 1994, 1998), and thus will only briefly summarise it here. We first placed each participant in the scanner, and aligned him or her on the bed relative to the orbitomeatal line. The participant then was given a thermoplastic face mask, nasal cannulae, and a vacuum mask. Following this, we used an orbiting rod source to obtain transmission measurements. For the scanning procedure itself, the participant inhaled ^{15}O-CO_2, mixed into room air. This mixture was delivered 15 s after the participant began to perform the task, and continued for another 60 s. The participants continued performing the tasks for an additional 12 s after the flow of ^{15}O-CO_2 was stopped. We waited approximately 10 min from the end of one block of trials before beginning another, which is enough time to ensure that any residual radioactivity was minimal. We used a GE Scanditronix PC4096 15-slice whole body tomograph, which produced contiguous slices 6.5 mm apart (centre-to-centre; the axial field was equal to 97.5 mm), and the axial resolution was 6.0 mm full width at half maximum (FWHM) (Rota-Kops, Herzog, Schmid, Holte, & Feinendegen, 1990). The participants received the ^{15}O-CO_2 at a concentration of 2800 MBq/L at a flow rate of 2 L/min; the measured peak count rate from the brain was 100,000–200,000 events/s.

RESULTS

Behavioural results

Table 1 presents the mean RTs and ERs for the four tasks, along with standard errors of the mean. As is evident, mean RTs were comparable across the four tasks, $p > .28$. The means ranged from 4006 ms to 4414 ms. However, the participants performed significantly faster the second time they performed the tasks, $F(1, 15) = 38.12, p < .0001$. Least square means comparisons revealed that this difference was significant for all four tasks, $p < .003$ in all cases. The analysis of ERs revealed that the tasks were not equally difficult, $F(3, 15) = 3.17, p < .04$. Least square means comparisons revealed two pairwise differences

TABLE 1

Mean response times in ms and percentage error rates with standard errors of the mean, for each of the four tasks, in each of the two replicates

Task	Replicate 1	Replicate 2	Task mean
Mean response times (ms)			
Resolution	4545 ± 429	3604 ± 315	4075 ± 275
Generation	4903 ± 369	3925 ± 342	4414 ± 263
Inspection	4424 ± 355	3588 ± 300	4006 ± 240
Transformation	4871 ± 372	3764 ± 317	4318 ± 260
Replicate mean	4686 ± 188	3720 ± 157	
Overall mean			4203
Percentage error rates (%)			
Resolution	18.4 ± 3.11	17.5 ± 2.80	18.0 ± 2.06
Generation	10.5 ± 2.39	7.9 ± 1.79	9.2 ± 2.49
Inspection	14.9 ± 3.66	9.3 ± 2.70	12.1 ± 2.29
Transformation	15.8 ± 3.65	12.5 ± 2.46	14.2 ± 2.18
Replicate mean	14.9 ± 1.62	11.8 ± 1.29	
Overall mean			13.4

between the tasks: the ER for the resolution task was higher than for either the generation ($p < .005$) or inspection tasks ($p = .05$). There were no other significant effects. In spite of the differences in accuracy between some tasks, ERs were sufficiently low in each case that we can have confidence that rCBF does reflect the processing used to accomplish the tasks. The pattern of means was the same in the two replications, Task × Replication $p > .80$.

We also performed correlational analyses on the ER and RT measures for each replicate of each task. Other than strong correlations between the first and second blocks for the same measure of the same task (which would be predicted if the task measurements are reliable), there were relatively few significant correlations (and none between RT and ER of the same task, which indicates that there were no speed–accuracy tradeoffs). The significant correlations, Bonferroni-corrected for multiple comparisons, were overwhelmingly with RT and with the second stimulus presentation of each task, as follows: Generation 2 RT/Inspection 2 RT; Generation 2 RT/Resolution 2 RT; Inspection 2 RT/Resolution 2 RT; Inspection 2 RT/Transformation 2 RT; Inspection 2 RT/Generation 2 ER; Resolution 2 RT/ Transformation 1 RT; Resolution 2 RT/Transformation 2 RT.

PET statistical analysis

The PET analyses were conducted using Statistical Parametric Mapping (SPM 99) software developed at the Wellcome Department of Imaging Neuroscience, Institute of Neurology, London, UK (see Friston, Frith, Liddle, & Frackowiak, 1991; Friston, Holmes, Worsley, Poline, Frith, & Frackowiak, 1995; Worsley,

Evans, Marrett, & Neelin, 1992). To correct for small amounts of head motion, the data were realigned relative to a single scan. They were then spatially normalised using the algorithms provided within the SPM 99 software package. Smoothing was 15 mm full width half maximum (FWHM). Using the "covariates only" option with proportional scaling around a normalised grand mean of 50 ml/min/100g, RTs and ERs were covaried with rCBF to produce 32 Z-score maps (one for each task/replicate/behavioural measure combination and for each of these a positive and negative covariate map). For each covariate analysis, a contrast was specified as either +1 or −1 in order to produce separate Z-score maps of rCBF voxel values that covaried positively or negatively with behavioural performance. A brain region was considered to be "positively correlated" with performance if increased blood flow in the region was associated with higher RTs or ERs; conversely, if increased blood flow in a region was associated with lower RTs or ERs, that brain region was considered to be "negatively correlated" with behavioural performance. In a covariate analysis, the SPM software essentially regresses an independent variable (in this case, voxel values representing normalised rCBF) onto a dependent variable (RTs or ERs). The voxels that fit the regression model (i.e., those where the relationship between rCBF and behavioural performance is significant across participants) appear on the Z-score map, where each voxel is accompanied by a Z-score for the contrast. Consistent with previous reports (Kosslyn et al., 1998, 1999) Z-scores of 3.09 or above were considered to be significant ($p = .001$, uncorrected). Scores on the Raven's Advanced Progressive Matrices test were included in the analysis as a "covariate of no interest", thereby removing the contribution of this measure.

The covariate analysis allowed us to identify 45 ROIs that would later be further examined in a forward stepwise regression analysis. Using software developed at the Massachusetts General Hospital PET laboratory, running on a platform designed by Advanced Visual Systems (AVS, Waltham, MA), ROIs were traced around the 45 points of peak rCBF identified in the covariates analysis. Depending on the size, in voxels, of the area initially discovered in the covariate analysis, the ROI was traced with a radius of either 6 mm (for brain areas that were smaller than 100 voxels in the covariate analysis) or 10 mm (for brain areas larger than 100 voxels upon initial identification). We identified 24 areas as covarying with RTs or ERs when a task was first performed (Replicate 1), and 21 such areas when a task was performed a second time (Replicate 2). We extracted values of mean rCBF for each of the regions.

For the stepwise regression analyses, we entered mean rCBF from all ROIs associated with Replicate 1 of any task as independent variables. The same procedure was repeated for Replicate 2. Eight separate regression analyses were conducted for each of the two replicates (for each of the combinations of the four tasks and two behavioural measures). Using version 5.0 of the Statview program for the Macintosh (SAS Institute, Cary, NC), we performed forward stepwise regressions.

PET results

Variations in four dependent variables (Resolution RT, Replicate 1; Resolution ER, Replicate 1; Transformation ER, Replicate 1; and Resolution ER, Replicate 2) were not predicted by any variable entered into the stepwise regression. Variations in the other 12 dependent variables were predicted by between one and six independent variables (ROIs). The total variance explained for each dependent variable that was predicted by at least one independent variable ranged between 68% to 95%. This result is consistent with that of Kosslyn et al. (1996), who found that 88% of the variance in performance (as measured by RTs) was accounted for by rCBF in three brain areas. Table 2 lists the predictors associated with each of the dependent variables (each dependent variable is a Task/Replicate/Behavioural measure combination) as well as the percentage of variance explained by each variable.

Figure 2 graphically summarises three aspects of the results. First, it shows the Talairach and Tournoux coordinates of each area in which variations in rCBF (over participants) accounted for variations in performance. Second, it illustrates the brain areas in which variations in rCBF (over participants) predicted performance in more than one task, as indicated by the overlap between circles. Third, it shows, for each area, whether the correlation was positive (higher rCBF = higher RT or ER) or negative (higher rCBF = lower RT or ER); brain areas that are negatively correlated with behavioural measures are preceded by a minus sign (−) in the figure.

Consider now the results for each task. First, variations in performance of the resolution task (Replicate 2) were driven by three areas, which accounted for 85.9% of the variance in RTs (the ERs in this task were not predicted by any brain regions). Two of the three areas were uniquely associated with performance of this task, the orbitofrontal gyrus and a region of the occipito-parietal sulcus. The third area, the medial frontal gyrus, was also associated with performance in the transformation task. Variations in performance of this task were not related to rCBF in primary or secondary visual cortex.

Second, variations in performance of the generation task were accounted for by variations in rCBF of 12 different areas, 4 of which also predicted variations in performance of other tasks. Perhaps most interesting, variations in performance of this task were predicted by three areas that also predicted variations in performance of the inspection task. This finding is intriguing because it is not intuitively obvious that the task of melding an image with a percept draws on processes also used to parse a character into segments and count them. Nevertheless, performance of the generation task clearly relied mostly on distinct processes, including ones that are implemented in Area 18 and middle occipital gyrus, near the border of Areas 18 and 19.

Third, variations in performance of the inspection task were predicted by variations in 11 areas, 7 of which were unique to this task. One of these areas

TABLE 2
Results of the stepwise forward multiple regression analyses

Step	Area	Talairach			% var. explained
Resolution 1 RT [model: n.s., $F < 1$]					
Generation 1 RT [model: $F = 10.01$, $p = .001$]					
Step 1	Brain stem	17	−19	−8	51.1
Step 2	Medial frontal	−4	55	18	20.4
Total					71.5
Inspection 1 RT [model: $F = 19.27$, $p < .0001$]					
Step 1	Medial frontal (9/10)	6	61	31	57.2
Step 2	Anterior cingulate (32)	1	35	30	17.6
Total					74.8
Transformation 1 RT [model: $F = 5.29$, $p = .02$]					
Step 1	Occ. temp. jct. (19/39)	43	−83	16	44.8
Step 2	Occ. par. sulcus	22	−71	19	34.8
Total					79.6
Resolution 1 ER [model: n.s., $F < 1$]					
Generation 1 ER [model: $F = 21.43$, $p < .0001$]					
Step 1	Caudate	3	4	12	42.0
Step 2	Occ. par. sulcus	22	−71	19	16.1
Step 3	Area 18	18	−73	3	21.4
Step 4	Medial frontal (9)	6	61	31	6.8
Step 5	Middle occ. (18/19)	−29	−83	22	7.2
Total					93.5
Inspection 1 ER [model: $F = 28.3$, $p < .0001$]					
Step 1	Transver. temp. (41/42)	34	−29	18	69.4
Step 2	Thalamus	−3	−13	6	18.2
Total					87.6
Transformation 1 ER [model: n.s., $F = 1.1$, $p > .32$]					
Resolution 2 RT [model: $F = 16.78$, $p < .0001$]					
Step 1	Medial frontal (10)	−13	61	−9	57.8
Step 2	Occ. par. sulcus	−18	−69	19	21.2
Step 3	Orbitofrontal gyrus	1	51	−12	6.9
Total					85.9
Generation 2 RT [model: $F = 15.93$, $p < .0003$]					
Step 1	Medial frontal (8)	−3	45	37	71.0
Total					71.0
Inspection 2 RT [model $F = 19.26$, $p = .0002$]					
Step 1	Medial frontal (8)	−3	45	37	37.2
Step 2	Area 19	−40	−75	6	16.4
Step 3	Insula	34	20	4	22.2
Step 4	Hippocampus	31	−32	−2	8.1
Step 5	Area 18	12	−77	24	7.0
Step 6	Thalamus	3	−11	6	3.5
Total					94.4
Transformation 2 RT [model: $F = 14.11$, $p = .0006$]					
Step 1	Medial frontal (10)	−13	61	−9	68.5
Total					68.5

(Continued overleaf)

TABLE 2
(Continued)

Step	Area	Talairach			% var. explained
Resolution 2 ER [model: n.s., $F < 1$]					
Generation 2 ER [model: $F = 21.3$, $p < .0001$]					
Step 1	Occ. par. sulcus	−18	−71	21	51.0
Step 2	Thalamus	3	−11	6	15.6
Step 3	Occ. par. sulcus	−18	−73	19	9.2
Step 4	Anterior cingulate (32)	3	28	31	15.6
Total					91.4
Inspection 2 ER [model: $F = 20.5$, $p < .0001$]					
Step 1	Area 18	−41	−91	6	68.5
Step 2	Hippocampus	31	−32	−2	15.2
Total					83.7
Transformation 2 ER [model: $F = 12.75$, $p = .0004$]					
Step 1	Area 18	−41	−91	6	48.1
Step 2	Posterior cingulate	6	−54	22	18.0
Step 3	Medial frontal (8)	10	45	34	16.2
Total					82.3

Results for each of the 16 independent variables are presented separately. For each independent variable (e.g., Resolution 1 RT, which is the response time for the first replicate of the resolution task), the results for the entire model are first presented, followed by the brain areas that predict performance, in the order in which they entered the equation. Brodmann's Areas, if available, are in parentheses. In addition, we provide Talairach coordinates (Talairach & Tournoux, 1988) of the regions, and the total percentage of variance explained.

was surprising at first glance: the transverse temporal gyrus (the primary auditory region). The positive correlation between performance and rCBF (lower rCBF, lower ER) may be due to transmodal inhibition: as participants become involved in a visual task that requires a high degree of visual attention, as would be expected in the inspection task, auditory processes are inhibited. As noted earlier, some of the variation in performance of this task was also accounted for by variations in the same areas that predicted performance in the generation task.

Finally, performance in the transformation task was predicted by variations in rCBF in six brain areas, three of which predicted performance only in this task. The transformation task was the only one that was predicted by variations in areas that also predicted performance in each of the other tasks. It is not intuitively obvious that the transformation task would draw on processes used in each of the other three tasks.

Several aspects of the results are worth particular attention. Performance in two of the tasks (inspection and transformation) was predicted by variations in rCBF in the same part of Area 18. This is interesting because Area 18 is

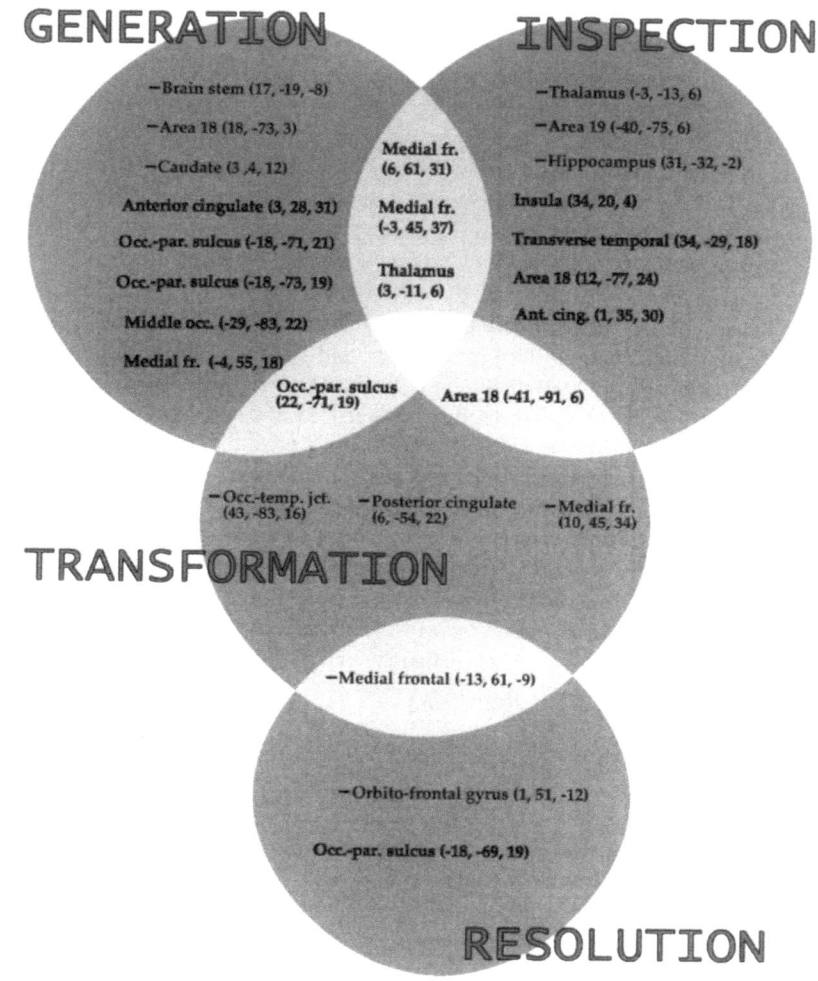

Figure 2. A Venn diagram illustrating the brain regions (with their Talairach & Tournoux coordinates) that predicted performance in each of the four tasks. Regions associated with any measure of performance in either replicate are shown within the circle representing that task. Note that although variations in performance of the tasks are largely predicted by independent areas of the brain, there is also some partial overlap. Negative correlations with behavioural measures (lower RT or ER = greater rCBF) are preceded by a minus sign (−). The first coordinate indicates position on the X axis, with negative values indexing the left cerebral hemisphere and positive values indexing the right cerebral hemisphere.

topographically mapped, and thus represents information in a "depictive" format. Variations in rCBF of another portion of Area 18 also accounted for performance in the generation task.

In addition, rCBF in portions of the occipito-parietal sulcus accounted for performance in three of the four tasks (all except inspection), but the left side predicted performance in the generation and resolution tasks and the right side predicted performance in the generation and transformation tasks.

Moreover, the sheer number of areas that predict behaviour lines up with the complexity of the task: The simplest task was the resolution task, which involves generating a single letter and judging two portions of it; the next most complicated task was rotation, which added one operation (rotation) to the resolution task but reduced the difficulty of the comparison *per se*; next was inspection, which involved not only generating the letter, but decomposing it into segments and then counting them in the key wedges; and finally was generation, which involves encoding the printed letter and adding to it the imaged letter, then comparing the combined overlapping pattern in the two key wedges. This ordering cannot be ascribed to differences in "difficulty": The participants performed the generation task best, and resolution worst. There are two factors that contribute to overall difficulty when performing a task—the number of operations, and the difficulty of each operation; the RTs and ERs appear to reflect the difficulty of the rate-limiting steps, not the complexity of overall processing *per se*.

And lastly, although most of these areas were unique to one task, about a quarter of them were shared; specifically, rCBF in a total of 26 areas predicted performance and 20 of these areas predicted performance only in a single task.

DISCUSSION

The most fundamental finding of this study was that most of the brain areas that predicted performance were associated with only one task, thus demonstrating that the tasks tap largely independent components of mental imagery. In all cases, variations in rCBF of at least one brain area predicted performance only in one of the tasks. However, we also found substantial sharing of underlying processes, as demonstrated by the overlap in regions that predict performance in the tasks. Thus, we have evidence that some processes drawn upon by the different tasks are shared, but most are distinct.

The key shared areas were in occipito-parietal sulcus (portions of which were activated in all except the inspection task), the medial frontal cortex (portions of which were activated in all tasks), and Area 18 (portions of which were activated in all but the resolution task). The occipito-parietal sulcus is probably involved in spatial representation, which is crucial to perform the comparison between wedges. The medial frontal cortex, which has connections to primary motor cortex and the parietal lobe, as well as to the basal ganglia and anterior cingulate gyrus, may be an integrative region involved in planning or setting up sequences (cf. Tanji, 2001). This region may mediate between attentional processes and action planning. And Area 18 is involved in representing the spatial layout of surfaces, which plays an important role in many forms of imagery (Kosslyn, Ganis, & Thompson, 2001; Thompson & Kosslyn, 2000).

The intercorrelations between measures of behavioural performance, specifically between the RTs in the second replicate of each task, suggest that as the participants become more practised, more general skills (not task-specific) may become more important in setting a rate-limiting step. Some of this variance might be subsumed by the regions illustrated in the common areas of the Venn diagram in Figure 2. However, we cannot address this question in detail; because of constraints on the number of scans we could administer to each participant, we could not collect data for a more general baseline condition that would share many of the same processes as these tasks and would serve as a "common denominator" for them. Nevertheless, both the PET results and behavioural correlations, particularly with respect to the first block of each task, suggest that the tasks were largely independent, with variations in performance arising from the operation of distinct neural mechanisms.

The unique areas were distributed widely in the brain. Some were surprising, such as the caudate and brain stem (for the generation task). We will not attempt to invent post hoc accounts for why variations in rCBF in these particular areas predicted variations in performance in the different tasks.

In addition, we found both positive and negative correlations. Positive correlations indicate that increased activation in an area was associated with poorer performance, whereas negative correlations indicate that increased activation was associated with better performance. The negative correlations are easy to explain: More vigorous brain activation results in faster and more accurate processing. But what about the positive correlations? We suggest two possible interpretations: On the one hand, perhaps people who are very good at some processes have become so well practised that they perform them with little effort. By analogy, a marathon runner can run a mile with less effort than a sedentary neuroscientist. Thus, it is possible that the positive correlations pick out areas that implement highly practised processes for some people. For those people, relatively little rCBF would occur when they perform very well. On the other hand, there may be multiple strategies for performing each task, and some are more efficient than others. If a participant adopts one particular strategy, one set of areas will be active—and if he or she adopts another strategy, another set of areas will be active. If so, then the positive correlations may indicate areas that are drawn upon by less efficient strategies, which require more cognitive work to accomplish.

It is also of interest to note that most negative correlations are in right-hemisphere areas, which may suggest that the processes carried out in this hemisphere are more effective than those in the left hemisphere. That is, more effort (reflected by greater rCBF) pays off by producing better performance. The use of right-hemisphere processes may suggest that "coordinate" spatial relations are used, which would be more useful than "categorical" spatial relations (such as "next to" or "above"; see Chabris & Kosslyn, 1998); such right-hemisphere activity may also suggest that representations of specific exemplars (Kosslyn, 1987) are used. Both coordinate spatial relations and representations of exemplar shapes would be useful for the judgements required in our tasks.

Perhaps the most striking aspect of the results is how far they deviated from our predictions. These predictions were all rooted in the results of previous studies, which relied on the subtractive logic. In the light of hindsight, this was probably an error: We should not expect the same areas to be identified in the two types of analyses. First, in a sense, the subtraction logic is the antithesis of the correlational logic: Individual variability in a subtraction design decreases the chance of observing a statistically reliable effect in a group design, whereas the opposite holds for a correlational design (assuming that the individual variability is correlated with the behavioural measure of interest). For instance, when there is wide variation in levels of activation the mean may not be significantly above threshold (because of the large variance), and yet the variations may correlate with performance and be revealed by a correlational design. Second, some of the areas that are activated more than baseline in the standard subtraction designs may implement "minimally sufficient" processes; if so, then even if they are active, variations in activation will not predict performance. In this case, the lack of a correlation with behaviour would reveal something about the function of an area that could not be inferred from using the subtraction logic alone.

The present research represents one of the first attempts to use the regression approach to study the relation among several tasks (cf. Ng, Bullmore, Zubicaray, Cooper, Suckling, & Williams, 2001). This is only an initial, rather modest, step. It is clear, however, that this approach holds promise of providing new insights into how the brain gives rise to performance.

PrEview proof published online May 2004

REFERENCES

Aguirre, G. K., Detre, J. A., Zarahn, E., & Alsop, D. C. (2002). Experimental design and the relative sensitivity of BOLD and perfusion MRI. *NeuroImage, 15,* 488–500.

Behrmann, M., Moscovitch, M., & Winocur, G. (1994). Intact visual imagery and impaired visual perception in a patient with visual agnosia. *Journal of Experimental Psychology: Human Perception and Performance, 20,* 1068–1087.

Bisiach, E., & Luzzatti, C. (1978). Unilateral neglect of representational space. *Cortex, 14,* 129–133.

Boring, E. G. (1950). *A history of experimental psychology* (2nd ed.). New York: Appleton-Century-Crofts.

Chabris, C. F., & Kosslyn, S. M. (1998). How do the cerebral hemispheres contribute to encoding spatial relations? *Current Directions in Psychological Science, 7,* 8–14.

Cohen J. D., MacWhinney B., Flatt M., & Provost J. (1993). PsyScope: A new graphic interactive environment for designing psychology experiments. *Behavioral Research Methods, Instruments and Computers, 25,* 257–271.

Cohen, M. S., Kosslyn, S. M., Breiter, H. C., DiGirolamo, G. J., Thompson, W. L., Bookheimer, S. Y., Belliveau, J. W., & Rosen, B. R. (1996). Changes in cortical activity during mental rotation: A mapping study using functional MRI. *Brain, 119,* 89–100.

Detre, J. A., & Wang, J. (2002). Technical aspects and utility of fMRI using BOLD and ASL. *Clinical Neurophysiology, 113,* 621–634.

Duncan, J., Seitz, R. J., Kolodny, J., Bor, D., Herzog, H., Ahmed, A., Newell, F. N., & Emslie, H. (2000). A neural basis for general intelligence. *Science, 289,* 457–460.

Farah, M. J. (1984). The neurological basis of mental imagery: A componential analysis. *Cognition, 18,* 245–272.

Farah, M. J. (2000). The neural bases of mental imagery. In M. S. Gazzaniga (Ed.), *The cognitive neurosciences* (2nd ed., pp. 965–974). Cambridge, MA: MIT Press.

Friston, K. J., Frith, C. D., Liddle, P. F., & Frackowiak, R. S. J. (1991). Comparing functional (PET) images: The assessment of significant changes. *Journal of Cerebral Blood Flow and Metabolism, 11,* 690–699.

Friston, K. J., Holmes, A. P., Worsley, K. J., Poline, J. B., Frith, C. D., & Frackowiak, R. S. J. (1995). Statistical parametric maps in functional imaging: A general approach: *Human Brain Mapping, 2,* 189–210.

Kandel, E. R., & Squire, L. R. (2000). Neuroscience: Breaking down scientific barriers to the study of brain and mind. *Science, 290,* 1113–1120.

Kosslyn, S. M. (1987). Seeing and imagining in the cerebral hemispheres: A computational approach. *Psychological Review, 94,* 148–175.

Kosslyn, S. M. (1999). If neuroimaging is the answer, what is the question? *Philosophical Transactions of the Royal Society, London B, 354,* 1283–1294.

Kosslyn, S. M., Alpert, N. M., Thompson, W. L., Chabris, C. F., Rauch, S. L., & Anderson, A. K. (1994). Identifying objects seen from different viewpoints: A PET investigation. *Brain, 117,* 1055–1071.

Kosslyn, S. M., Brunn, J. L., Cave, K. R., & Wallach, R. W. (1984). Individual differences in visual imagery: A computational analysis. *Cognition, 18,* 195–243.

Kosslyn, S. M., DiGirolamo, G., Thompson, W. L., & Alpert, N. M. (1998). Mental rotation of objects versus hands: Neural mechanisms revealed by positron emission tomography. *Psychophysiology, 35,* 151–161.

Kosslyn, S. M., Ganis, G., & Thompson, W. L. (2001). Neural foundations of imagery. *Nature Reviews: Neuroscience, 2,* 635–642.

Kosslyn, S. M., Pascual-Leone, A., Felician, O., Camposano, S., Keenan, J. P., Thompson, W. L., Ganis, G., Sukel, K. E., & Alpert, N. M. (1999). The role of area 17 in visual imagery: Convergent evidence from PET and rTMS. *Science, 284,* 167–170.

Kosslyn, S. M., & Plomin, R. (2001). Towards a neurocognitive genetics: Goals and issues. In D. Dougherty, S. L. Rauch, & J. F. Rosenbaum (Eds.), *Psychiatric neuroimaging research: Contemporary strategies* (pp. 383–402). Washington, DC: American Psychiatric Press.

Kosslyn, S. M., Thompson, W. L., & Alpert, N. M. (1997). Neural systems shared by visual imagery and visual perception: A positron emission tomography study. *NeuroImage, 6,* 320–334.

Kosslyn, S. M., Thompson, W. L., Kim, I. J., Rauch, S. L., & Alpert, N. M. (1996). Individual differences in cerebral blood flow in area 17 predict the time to evaluate visualized letters. *Journal of Cognitive Neuroscience, 8,* 78–82.

Külpe, O. (1895). *Outlines of psychology.* New York: Macmillan.

Luce, R. D. (1986). *Response times: Their role in inferring elementary mental organization.* New York: Oxford University Press.

Mast, F. W., & Kosslyn, S. M. (2002). Visual mental images can be ambiguous: Insights from individual differences in spatial transformation abilities. *Cognition, 86,* 57–70.

Mellet, E., Petit, L., Mazoyer, B., Denis, M., & Tzourio, N. (1998). Reopening the mental imagery debate: Lessons from functional anatomy. *NeuroImage, 8,* 129–139.

Ng, V. W., Bullmore, E. T., Zubicaray, G. I., Cooper, A., Suckling, J., & Williams, S. C. (2001). Identifying rate-limiting nodes in large-scale cortical networks for visuospatial processing: An illustration using fMRI. *Journal of Cognitive Neuroscience, 13,* 537–545.

Raven, J., Raven, J. C., & Court, J. H. (1998). *Manual for Raven's Progressive Matrices and Vocabulary Scales: Section 4, Advanced Progressive Matrices, Sets I and II.* Oxford, UK: Oxford Psychologists Press.

Rota-Kops, E., Herzog, H. H., Schmid, A., Holte, S., & Feinendegen, L. E. (1990). Performance characteristics of an eight-ring whole body PET scanner. *Journal of Computer Assisted Tomography, 14,* 437–445.

Smith, E. E., & Jonides, J. (1997). Working memory: A view from neuro-imaging. *Cognitive Psychology, 33,* 5–42.

Talairach, J., & Tournoux, P. (1988). *Co-planar stereotaxic atlas of the human brain* (M. Rayport, Trans.). New York: Thieme.

Tanji, J. (2001). Sequential organization of multiple movements: Involvement of cortical motor areas. *Annual Review of Neuroscience, 24,* 631–651.

Thompson, W. L., & Kosslyn, S. M. (2000). Neural systems activated during visual mental imagery: A review and meta-analyses. In A. W. Toga & J. C. Mazziotta (Eds.), *Brain mapping: The systems* (pp. 535–560). San Diego, CA: Academic Press.

Woodworth, R. S. (1938). *Experimental psychology.* New York: Henry Holt.

Worsley, K. J., Evans, A. C., Marrett, S., & Neelin, P. (1992) A three-dimensional statistical analysis for rCBF activation studies in human brain. *Journal of Cerebral Blood Flow and Metabolism, 12,* 900–918.

EUROPEAN JOURNAL OF COGNITIVE PSYCHOLOGY, 2004, *16* (5), 717–728

Mental rotation and the parietal question in functional neuroimaging: A discussion of two views

Vinoth Jagaroo

Department of Psychiatry and the Behavioral Neuroscience Program, Boston University School of Medicine, and Department of Communication Sciences and Disorders, Emerson College, Boston

This review addresses the meaning of parietal activation in functional imaging studies of mental rotation. It focuses on parietal activity with primary reference to the 3-D cube array task. Key functional imaging studies of mental rotation are surveyed to bring forth two current perspectives on the meaning of parietal activation: (1) a dominant mechanism for whole-object coordinate transformation which accounts for the parietal-based "bulk" of mental rotation, and (2) various visuospatial parietal mechanisms including but not dominated by a coordinate transformational mechanism, which only together account for the strength of parietal activation. The centrality of coordinate transformations, particularly to the first perspective, is highlighted. Many basic questions about rotational coordinate mechanics are posed—suggesting some specific issues for future work on functional imaging of mental rotation. This article simply attempts to lay out the dominant perspectives of parietal activation in mental rotation, how they have gained validity, and the complications they face when discrete computations on which they hinge, are factored in.

Together with the salience of functional imaging results on mental rotation has come an array of new questions. These have made tenuous any interpretation of clear associations between mental rotation processes and the neural systems underlying these processes. Disparities among results of functional imaging studies examining very similar mental rotation tasks have also complicated the picture. Questions arising from functional imaging studies have opened new discussions and prompted caution about tempting associations between cognitive processes of mental rotation and the neural systems that appear to underlie them (see Just, Carpenter, Keller, Emery, Zajac, & Thulborn, 2001; Kosslyn, 1999).

Correspondence should be addressed to Vinoth Jagaroo, Dept. of Communication Sciences & Disorders, Emerson College, 216 Tremont Street, 9th Floor, Boston, MA 02116, USA. Email: jagaroo@bu.edu

http://www.tandf.co.uk/journals/pp/09541446.html   DOI: 10.1080/09541440340000466

A generally consistent finding among functional imaging studies of mental rotation has been activation in regions of the posterior parietal cortex (PPC), albeit differentially and among other cortical areas activated: Positron emission tomography has shown PPC activation during mental rotation of alphanumeric and body-part objects (Alivisatos & Petrides, 1997; Bonda, Petrides, Frey, & Evans, 1995; Harris, Egan, Sonkkila, Tochon-Danguy, Paxinos, & Watson, 2000; Vingerhoets, Santens, van Laere, LaHorte, Dierckx, & de Reuck, 2001). Posterior parietal cortex activation during mental rotation of the Shepard and Metzler (1971) 3-D cube array task or similar tasks has been widely demonstrated by functional MRI (Barnes et al., 2000; Carpenter, Just, Keller, Eddy, & Thulborn, 1999; Cohen et al., 1996; Gauthier, Hayward, Tarr, Anderson, Skudlarski, & Gore, 2002; Jordan, Heinze, Lutz, Kanowski, & Jancke, 2001; Ng, Bullmore, Zubicaray, Cooper, Suckling, & Williams, 2001; Richter, Ugurbil, Georgopoulo, & Kim, 1997; Tagaris, Kim, Strupp, Andersen, Ugurbil, & Georgopoulos, 1996; Thomsen et al., 2000; Vanrie, Béatse, Wagemans Sunaert, & van Hecke, 2002; Zacks, Rypma, Gabrieli, Tversky, & Glover, 1999). These findings have been consistent with the PPC role in high-level spatial processes such as transformation of spatial coordinates and the representation of spatial reference frames as suggested by neurophysiological studies on non-human primates (Andersen, Snyder, Batista, Buneo, & Cohen, 1998; Andersen, Snyder, Li, & Stricanne, 1993; Snyder, Batista, & Andersen, 2000). In attempting to layout a neural mechanism for mental rotation, much discussion in functional imaging studies has focused on the precise role of the PPC in this cognitive operation. A preponderance of studies have utilised the Shepard and Metzler 3-D cube array shape rotation task (hereafter referred to as the shape rotation test or task). As a powerful, high fidelity paradigm that has long challenged cognitive science, the shape rotation task has, quite appreciatively, been a prime target of functional imaging studies of mental rotation. Based on differing functional activation patterns and differing interpretations of supporting theoretical data, these functional imaging studies have also presented two interpretations of parietal activation and hence different notions about parietal neural activity in mental rotation.

This issue is not whether numerous cortical areas spanning prefrontal, parietal and occipitotemporal areas are involved in performance of the shape rotation test. There is general substantiation of a widespread cortical network in mental rotation, along the lines proposed by Cohen et al. (for example, see Vingerhoets et al., 2001), although questions about the extent of its hemispheric lateralisation remain. Also, the functional imaging discussions on the roles the motor cortex (Kosslyn, Thompson, Wraga, & Alpert, 2001; Richter et al., 2000) and primary visual cortex (Klein, Paradis, Poline, Kosslyn, & Le Bihan, 2000; Mellet, Tzourio-Mazoyer, Bricogne, Mazoyer, Kosslyn, & Denis, 2000) in mental imagery or rotation are separate from the parietal question. The parietal question is about the meaning of parietal activation, among a network of neural nodes activated, during mental rotation.

THE POSTERIOR PARIETAL CORTEX AND ROTATION PER SE

Bilateral activity in the superior parietal lobule and activity within the left intraparietal sulcus and inferior parietal lobule when subjects mentally rotated photographs of a human hand, was shown by Bonda et al. (1995). This activation was interpreted as a reflection of specialised parietal function in the transformation of spatial parameters of body projections. Alivisatos and Petrides (1997) indicated that during 2-D alphanumeric mental rotation, activity in the left inferior parietal region extending into the posterosuperior parietal cortex, was specific to these parietal regions (particularly the latter) and that this was indicative of the demands of actual rotation. Booth, MacWhinney, Thulborn, Sacco, Voyvodic, and Feldman (2000) in an fMRI study using the same alphanumeric 2-D rotation task as Alivisatos and Petrides, concluded that the superior parietal area is "directly involved in the rotation of visual stimuli" (p. 164). In the fMRI study by Cohen et al. (1996) using the shape rotation task, the activation of the superior parietal lobule (SPL) particularly BA 7, was interpreted as showing that "the bulk of the computation for mental rotation" (p. 97) is performed by the SPL. In the time-resolved fMRI study by Richter et al. (1997), the functional activation during the shape rotation task suggested parietal activity during the full length of mental rotation operations. The activity was seen as varying with reaction time and not with between-trial constancies, which suggested parietal involvement in "the very act of mental rotation" (p. 3697).

In these studies supporting the view that parietal activation represents the locus of the core or essential act of mental rotation, there is an implicit and necessary notion about the nature of this rotation. Rotation of an object or its spatiotopic coordinates occurs around an axis or along the path of a vector. The rotation may occur along a canonical or orthogonal plane. It is this (1) rotation of an object, its defining coordinates, or its fundamental axes, or (2) movement around a point to which an axis is attached, or (3) rotation along an orthogonal trajectory, that is reflected in the functional images of parietal activity. Cohen et al., for example, embrace this view as a part of a plausible mechanism for mental rotation, by referring to a solid object with three-dimensional extents that is rotated in solid and singular form by the SPL. This notion is consistent with the theory that speed of rotation bears no simple correlation with stimulus complexity (see Shepard & Cooper, 1986) and it is also consistent with the primacy of global imagery under appropriate circumstances (see Kosslyn, 1980, 1994). It can also be rationalised by the view that a specialised neural mechanism that performs general directional and coordinate transformations is the mechanism utilised in mental rotation (see de'Sperati, 1999). While the PPC holds specialised cell fields for different sensory signals, direction of attention, and motor planning (Andersen, Asanuma, Essick, & Siegel, 1990; Blatt, Andersen, & Stoner, 1990), it also uses a common coordinate frame for sensory signals (Andersen et al., 1998). A shared PPC population of neurons will perform a set of coordinate transformations when sampled in one way and will perform a different set of transformations when sampled in another way. Nevertheless, it is the same population of neurons performing these different coordinate transformations. (There is a consistency between this description of parietal rotational neural mechanisms and the fMRI finding by Barnes et al. (2000) on a linear transformation task and the shape rotation task. Both tasks produced increases in fMRI activation in BA 19.) It is also conceivable that in mental rotation, an ensemble of parietal neurons will fire directionally and produce a weighted neuronal population vector that rotates with imagined movement. This has been demonstrated with directionally tuned motor cortex neurons involved with physical movement requiring imagined transformations (Georgopoulos, 2000; Georgopoulos, Lurito, Petrides, Schwartz, & Massey, 1989). A parietal neuronal population vector acting in this fashion would firmly embody the notion of whole-object configural rotation or the "very act" of rotation.

ROTATION AS A FUNCTION OF SEVERAL "NONDOMINANT" VISUOSPATIAL TRANSFORMATIONS

Diverging from the above viewpoint, functional imaging studies of mental rotation have also suggested another explanatory mechanism for PPC activation. The significant correlation between SPL fMRI activation intensity and proportion of errors on the shape rotation task, as shown by Tagaris et al. (1996), was considered to be due to several possible factors, for example, the SPL's encoding of the stimulus objects; incorrect comparison of identical and mirror-reversed 3-D cube arrays; and errors in actual rotation of the stimulus object. Harris et al. (2000), in a PET study of mental rotation using alphanumeric characters, associated rotational task demand only with the right posterior parietal area (centring on the intraparietal sulcus). However, mental rotation, the authors suggested, involves just some of the variety of spatial transformations that the right PPC underlies. Parietal activation during rotation could also be reflective of the PPC's involvement in directing eye movements at the stimulus object. Harris et al. cited results from numerous neurophysiological studies (for example, Colby, Duhamel, & Goldberg, 1993; Gnadt & Andersen, 1988; Sakata, Taira, Mine, & Murata, 1992) as support for the claim that the PPC maps saccadic information into a coordinate system; specifically, they note that neurons in the PPC dynamically and continuously update location, direction, speed of motion, and changes in the orientation of objects. It was suggested that a part of this complex of visuospatial functionality constitutes the visuospatial transformations involved in mental rotation and this accounts for the intensity of parietal activation in mental rotation (referring more specifically to the right intraparietal sulcus). A similar line of reasoning was adopted by Jordan et al. (2001) in explaining a finding of bilateral fMRI activation around the IPS, activation that was common to three mental rotation tasks including the shape rotation task. Mental representation and rotation in the IPS derives from IPS functions of receiving signals from the primary visual areas V1, V2, and V3 and generating 2-D and 3-D mental representations. These signals are then manipulated or explored by motor or mental means. This remains an "action oriented" form of representation. A further possibility, the authors speculate, has to do with the IPS's working memory processes for spatial targets. Comparison of target and model stimuli in mental rotation, necessary in some mental rotation tasks, will involve working memory for continuous update of performance. All these processes may be required for rotation and only collectively do they account for intensity and extent of the parietal activation.

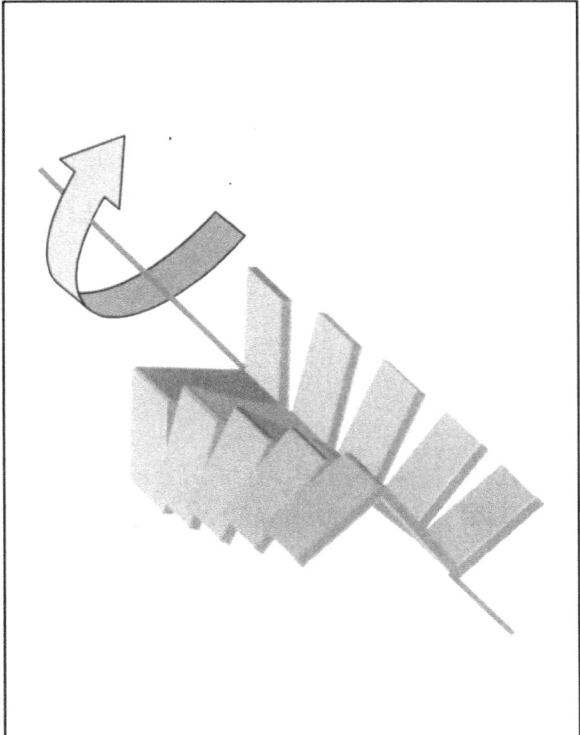

Figure 1. Schematic illustration of actual whole object rotation or coordinate transformation of an object that may account for the bulk of parietal activity. (A possible mechanism for this possibly dominant operation is a directionally tuned neuronal population vector.)

These multifunctional interpretations provide an equally compelling account of parietal activation. However, the difficulty of tying together parietal and extraparietal processes to articulate a fundamental act of rotation, inevitably makes such interpretations less appealing than the holistic dominant-rotation-factor perspective.

The two views on parietal activation do not discount the processes highlighted by each other. They merely place a different emphasis on relative degree to which these processes account for parietal activation in mental rotation. Figures 1 and 2 provide simple schematic illustrations of each of the two perspectives, respectively.

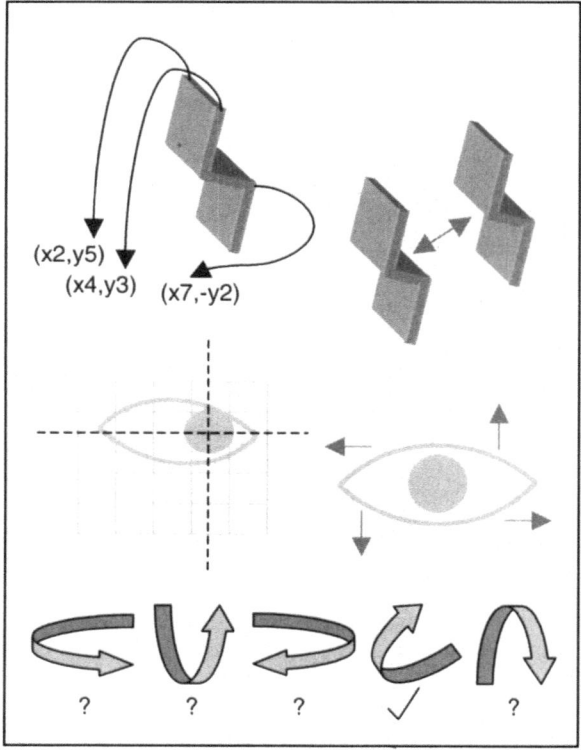

Figure 2.   Schematic illustration of some visuospatial operations and performance factors that may account for the strength of parietal activation. Actual rotation is merely one of these operations, and may not alone account for the strength of parietal activation. Some of these parietal visuospatial operations and performance factors are: object encoding, comparison of objects and errors in matching, working memory processes (parietal), rotation and rotational errors, directing and mapping saccadic movements, updating of parietal neurons (direction, motion, etc.), generation of mental images.

THE CRITICAL FACTOR OF COORDINATE TRANSFORMATIONS

The perspective of holistic parietal-based rotation centres firmly on the notion of a transformation of spatiotopic coordinates. Even findings of parietal event-related potentials in relation to angular disparity in mental rotation tasks have been cast within this framework of parietal-based coordinate transformation (Yoshino, Inoue, & Suzuki, 2000). The dynamics of coordinate computation and coordinate transformation underlie in some way or the other much of the discussion on parietal activation in mental rotation.

Carpenter et al. (1999) presented a "graded functional activation" model based on task demand. The model proposed that successive orientations and mental representations required across a greater rotational angle will require greater neuronal-computational resources. Increased parietal activation during wider rotational angles must therefore represent the increased parietal resources given to coordinate computational demands. Further distinctions on task demand and computational efficiency in the model proposed by Carpenter et al., were made by Ng et al. (2001). Ng et al. suggested that the superior parietal cortex was the site of activation most specific to the shape rotation task and indicative of the "rate limiting" node in the networks subserving the task. The task may be computationally demanding on the greater network but the slowest neural node (SPL in the case of shape rotation) reflects the extra demand the task makes on this node. A task that is computationally demanding will slow down the node because the node is probably working extra hard at the particular task (Ng, personal communication, 29 March 2002). The actual operation of "spatial transformations" in the shape rotation task, Ng et al. further suggested, would constitute the rate-limiting step of the task.

Gauthier et al. (2002) demonstrated fMRI activation differences in the SPL and IPL in relation to viewpoint (axial) differences in a 3-D rotation task. The vividness of axial effects prompted their suggestion that the transformation of coordinates in mental rotation may not be smooth and continuous. This perspective does not negate the notion of coordinate transformation along a trajectory. It merely raises the possibility that the mechanism may not always be fluent.

Resolving the components of parietal activation that are tied directly to coordinate computation and transformation is a critically important step in understanding parietal activation in mental rotation. There appear to be many possibilities for how parietal neuronal ensembles may format the coordinate transformation process. A rich spatiotopic encoding with minimal actual transformation, or minimal coordinate encoding and efficient rotational trajectories, may each produce the same degree of parietal activation. With such possibilities, it is obvious that both perspectives of parietal activation described by this paper can be affirmed—by considering individual differences in strategy.

However, the more fundamental question remains, that is, which of the two perspectives describes a natural or primary parietal mechanism for rotation if there is one?

CONCLUDING REMARKS

Many of the questions that can shed light on the meaning of parietal activation will perhaps best be able to do so only with further advances in temporal and structural resolution in functional imaging. As this process occurs, it will be useful to keep in mind some basic questions about computational possibilities in rotation. Consider the following.

Is parietal activity in mental rotation constituted by both a purely high-level motion trajectory operation and a separate spatiotopic structure which locks onto this trajectory? Or, is the interplay between these two systems so finely meshed such that it becomes unfeasible to parse them out in cognitive and functional imaging terms? Does the parietal cortex utilise an exclusive representational system for transformational trajectories? Or, as suggested by Senior et al. (1999), does the parietal cortex modulate visual cortex motion representation in a shared system for motion representation? Can motion representation mechanisms tune the trajectories for 3-D image transformation (as suggested by Kourtzi & Shiffrar, 1999)? Do they facilitate the jumps between successive views along the transformational gradient hence integrating the rotational sequence?

Is the vector trajectory for rotation always predetermined and firmly established? Alternately, does it develop only as each set of coordinates unfold (as in the case of representational momentum—see Hubbard, 1995)? The latter possibility would appear to be inconsistent with the deterministic view of neuronal-population-vector rotation (Georgopoulos, 2000; Georgopoulos et al., 1989) when the vector model is applied analogously to parietal transformations. More in phase with Hubbard's view of a stepwise trajectory development would be alternative views of neuronal population vector rotation such as that proposed by Cisek and Scott (1999). Here, a directionally tuned neuronal population vector starts rotating in the direction of movement. Neurons with broad directional tuning are then recruited during subsequent steps and they learn the required coordinate transformation by associating the stimulus cue with the direction reward. (Again, this is a model of neuronal population vector rotation in the motor cortex in response to physical rotation. It is applied as an analogy for parietal activity in mental rotation.) Either possibility, a predetermined trajectory or one that develops in a stepwise manner, may produce a similar degree of parietal activation in mental rotation.

What are some of the computational options involved with the multifunctional perspective of parietal activation? Is it possible that the activation may represent a kind of transformational dynamic that does not depend on a metric, canonical system for rotation? This would be an extreme interpretation of the perspective, but some computational models of mental rotation may agree: Beňušková and Eštok (1998), building on Dotsenko (1988) and Hopfield (1982), described a model for pattern recognition used within a mental rotation framework. In this model, the configuration of activity in a neuronal matrix at a given time represents the visual pattern. Gregson (1998) suggested that through "nonlinear multidimensional dynamics", patterns are created, erased and recreated at each instant. Eliminating a metric, canonical system for rotation, the model implies that mental rotation is the perceived phenomenon of a rapid succession of created, destroyed, and/or recreated images.

All these computational possibilities bear heavily on the enormous complexity in interpreting parietal activation in mental rotation. The strength and consistency of parietal activation leaves the compelling conclusion of a parietal locus for the "very act of mental rotation" (quoting Richter et al., 1997, p. 3697). When interpreted against coordinate frameworks for spatiotopic manipulation and directional trajectories, the very act of mental rotation often turns to an act of coordinate transformation. When the many possibilities for coordinate transformational processes are spelled out, the boundaries between the two perspectives of parietal activation can become blurred. Even within the dominant-rotation-factor perspective, a finer interpretation of parietal activation is likely to depend on which aspect of the coordinate-transformational process is emphasised.

Parietal processes in mental rotation alone pose a huge challenge to functional imaging in that they appear to constitute the core micromechanics of rotation. Clarifying the activation patterns elicited by the shape rotation test has thus far been a major focus in functional imaging studies of mental rotation. Tied to this pursuit is the challenge of interpreting discrete parietal operations in relation to rotational dynamics. Functional imaging of mental rotation will sooner or later have to map (1) neural nodes for general purpose spatiotopic transformations, (2) neural mechanisms which may achieve a rotational task without any dominant reliance on whole configural rotation, and (3) most challenging of all, the mapping of the interplay between these two larger systems in the many ways in which they could combine to perform the task.

PrEview proof published online May 2004

REFERENCES

Alivisatos, B., & Petrides, M. (1997). Functional activation of the human brain during mental rotation. *Neuropsychologia, 35,* 111–118.

Andersen, R. A., Asanuma, C., Essick, G., & Siegel, R. M. (1990). Corticocortical connections of anatomically and physiologically defined subdivisions within the inferior parietal lobule. *Journal of Comparative Neurology, 296,* 65–113.

Andersen, R. A., Snyder, L. H., Batista, A. P., Buneo, C. A., & Cohen, Y. E. (1998). Posterior parietal areas specialized for eye movements (LIP) and reach (PRR) using a common coordinate frame. In G. Bock & J. Goode (Eds.), *Sensory guidance of movement* (Novartis Foundation Symposium no. 218, pp. 109–122; Discussion, pp. 171–175). Chichester, UK: Wiley.

Andersen, R. A., Snyder, L. H., Li, C.-S., & Stricanne, B. (1993). Coordinate transformations in the representation of spatial information. *Current Opinion in Neurobiology, 3*, 171–176.

Barnes, J., Howard, R. J., Senior, C., Brammer, M., Bullmore, E. T., Simmons, A., Woodruff, P., & David, A. S. (2000). Cortical activity during rotational and linear transformations. *Neuropsychologia, 38*, 1148–1156.

Beňušková, L., & Eštok, S. (1998). Hypothetical neural mechanism that may play a role in mental rotation: An attractor neural network model. *Network: Computation in Neural Systems, 9*, 513–530.

Blatt, G., Andersen, R. A., & Stoner, G. (1990). Visual receptive field organization and cortico-cortical connections of area lip in the macaque. *Journal of Comparative Neurology, 299*, 421–445.

Bonda, E., Petrides, M., Frey, S., & Evans, A. (1995). Neural correlates of mental transformations of the body-in-space. *Proceedings of the National Academy of Sciences, USA, 92*, 11180–11184.

Booth, J. R., MacWhinney, B., Thulborn, K. R., Sacco, K., Voyvodic, J. T., & Feldman, H. M. (2000). Developmental and lesion effects in brain activation during sentence comprehension and mental rotation. *Developmental Neuropsychology, 18*, 139–169.

Carpenter, P., Just, M. A., Keller, T. A., Eddy, W., & Thulborn, K. (1999). Graded functional activation in the visuospatial system with the amount of task demand. *Journal of Cognitive Neuroscience, 11*, 9–24.

Cisek, P., & Scott, S. H. (1999). An alternative interpretation of population vector rotation in macaque motor cortex. *Neuroscience Letters, 272*, 1–4.

Cohen, M. S., Kosslyn, S. M., Breiter, H. C., DiGirolamo, G. J., Thompson, W. L., Anderson, A. K., et al. (1996). Changes in cortical activity during mental rotation: A mapping study using functional MRI. *Brain, 119*, 89–100.

Colby, C. L., Duhamel, J. R., & Goldberg, M. E. (1993). Ventral intraparietal area of the macaque: Anatomic location and visual response properties. *Journal of Neurophysiology, 69*, 902–914.

De'Sperati, C. (1999). Saccades to mentally rotated targets. *Experimental Brain Research, 126*, 563–577.

Dotsenko, V. S. (1988). Neural networks: Translation-, rotation-, and scale invariant patterns recognition. *Journal of Physics A: Mathematical and General, 21*, L783–787.

Gauthier, I., Hayward, W. G., Tarr, M. J., Anderson, A. W., Skudlarski, P., & Gore, J. C. (2002). BOLD activity during mental rotation and viewpoint-dependent object recognition. *Neuron, 34*, 161–171.

Georgopoulos, A. P. (2000). Cognition: Mental rotation (Perspectives: Images in neuroscience). *American Journal of Psychiatry, 157*, 695–696.

Georgopoulos, A. P., Lurito, J. P., Petrides, M., Schwartz, A. B., & Massey, J. T. (1989). Mental rotation of the neuronal population vector. *Science, 243*, 234–236.

Gnadt, J. W., & Andersen, R. A. (1988). Memory related motor planning activity in posterior parietal cortex of macaque. *Experimental Brain Research, 70*, 216–220.

Gregson, R. A. M. (1998). Confusing rotation-like operations in space, mind and brain. *British Journal of Mathematical and Statistical Psychology, 51*, 135–162.

Harris, I. M., Egan, G. F., Sonkkila, C., Tochon-Danguy, H., Paxinos, G., & Watson, J. D. G. (2000). Selective right parietal lobe activation during mental rotation. *Brain, 123*, 65–73.

Hopfield, J. J. (1982). Neural networks and physical systems with emergent collective computational abilities. *Proceedings of the National Academy of Sciences, USA, 79*, 2554–2558.

Hubbard, T. L. (1995). Environmental invariants in the representation of motion: Implied dynamics and representational momentum, gravity, friction and centripetal force. *Psychonomic Bulletin and Review, 2*, 322–338.

Jordan, K., Heinze, H.-J., Lutz, K., Kanowski, M., & Jancke, L. (2001). Cortical activations during mental rotation of different visual objects. *NeuroImage, 13*, 143–152.

Just, M. A., Carpenter, P., & Keller, T. A., Emery, L., Zajac, H., & Thulborn, K. R. (2001). Interdependence of nonoverlapping cortical systems in dual cognitive tasks. *NeuroImage, 14*, 417–426.

Klein, I., Paradis, A.-L., Poline, J.-B., Kosslyn, S. M., & Le Bihan, D. (2000). Transient activity in the human calcarine cortex during visual mental imagery: An event-related fMRI study. *Journal of Cognitive Neuroscience, 12*, 15–23.

Kosslyn, S. M. (1980). *Image and mind.* Cambridge, MA: Harvard University Press.

Kosslyn, S. M. (1994). *Image and brain: The resolution of the imagery debate.* Cambridge, MA: MIT Press.

Kosslyn, S. M. (1999). If neuroimaging is the answer, what is the question? *Philosophical Transactions of the Royal Society of London, Series B, 354*, 1283–1294.

Kosslyn, S. M., Thompson, W. L., Wraga, M., & Alpert, N. M. (2001). Imagining rotation by endogenous versus exogenous forces: Distinct neural mechanisms. *Neuroreport, 12*, 2519–2525.

Kourtzi, Z., & Shiffrar, M. (1999). The visual representation of three-dimensional, rotating objects. *Acta Psychologia, 102*, 265–292.

Mellet, E., Tzourio-Mazoyer, N., Bricogne, S., Mazoyer, B., Kosslyn, S. M., & Denis, M. (2000). Functional anatomy of high-resolution visual mental imagery. *Journal of Cognitive Neuroscience, 12*, 98–109.

Ng, V. W. K., Bullmore, E. T., de Zubicaray, G. I., Cooper, A., Suckling, J., & Williams, S. C. R. (2001). Identifying rate-limiting nodes in large-scale cortical networks for visuospatial processing: An illustration using fMRI. *Journal of Cognitive Neuroscience, 13*, 537–545.

Richter, W., Somorjai, R., Summers, R., Jarmasz, M., Menon, R. S., Gati, J. S., Georgopoulos, A. P., Tegeler, C., Ugurbil, K., & Kim, S.-G. (2000). Motor area activity during mental rotation studied by time-resolved single-trial fMRI. *Journal of Cognitive Neuroscience, 12*, 310–320.

Richter, W., Ugurbil, K., Georgopoulos, A., & Kim, S.-G. (1997). Time-resolved fMRI of mental rotation. *Neuroreport, 8*, 3697–3702.

Sakata, H., Taira, M., Mine, S., & Murata, A. (1992). Hand-movement-related neurons of the posterior parietal cortex of the monkey: Their role in the visual guidance of hand movements. In R. Caminiti, P. B. Johnson, & Y. Burnod (Eds.), *Control of arm movement in space* (pp. 185–198). Berlin: Springer-Verlag.

Senior, C., Barnes, J., Giampietro, V., Simmons, A., Bullmore, E. T., Brammer, M., et al. (1999). The functional neuroanatomy of implicit-motion perception or "representational momentum". *Current Biology, 10*, 16–22.

Shepard, R. N., & Cooper, L. A. (1986). *Mental images and their transformations.* Cambridge, MA: MIT Press.

Shepard, R. N., & Metzler, J. (1971). Mental rotation of three-dimensional objects. *Science, 171*, 701–703.

Snyder, L. H., Batista, A. P., & Andersen, R. A. (2000). Intention-related activity in the parietal cortex: A review. *Vision Research, 40*, 1433–1441.

Tagaris, A. G., Kim, S.-G., Strupp, J. P., Andersen, P., Ugurbil, K., & Georgopoulos, A. (1996). Quantitative relations between parietal activation and performance in mental rotation. *Neuroreport, 7*, 773–776.

Thomsen, T., Hugdahl, K., Ersland, L., Barndon, R., Lundervold, A., Smievoll, A. I., et al. (2000). Functional magnetic resonance imaging (fMRI) study of sex differences in a mental rotation task. *Medical Science Monitor, 6*, 1186–1196.

Vanrie, J., Béatse, E., Wagemans, J., Sunaert, S., & van Hecke, P. V. (2002). Mental rotation versus invariant features in object perception from diffferent viewpoints: An fMRI study. *Neuropsychologia, 40*, 917–930.

Vingerhoets, G., Santens, P., van Laere, K., LaHorte, P., Dierckx, R. A., & de Reuck, J. (2001). Regional brain activity during different paradigms of mental rotation in healthy volunteers: A positron emission tomography study. *NeuroImage, 13*, 381–391.

Yoshino, A., Inoue, M., & Suzuki, A. (2000). A topographic electrophysiologic study of mental rotation. *Cognitive Brain Research, 9*, 121–124.

Zacks, J., Rypma, B., Gabrieli, J. D. E., Tversky, B., & Glover, G. H. (1999). Imagined transformations of bodies: An fMRI investigation. *Neuropsychologia, 37*, 1029–1040.

EUROPEAN JOURNAL OF COGNITIVE PSYCHOLOGY, 2004, *16* (5), 729–752

Intermodal sensory image generation: An fMRI analysis

Marta Olivetti Belardinelli

ECONA and Department of Psychology, University of Rome "La Sapienza", Italy

Rosalia Di Matteo

Department of Clinical Sciences and Bio-images, University of Chieti "G. D'Annunzio", Italy

Cosimo Del Gratta

Department of Clinical Sciences and Bio-images and Institute of Advanced Biomedical Technologies, University of Chieti "G. D'Annunzio", and National Institute for the Physics of Matter, Research Unit of L'Aquila, Italy

Andrea De Nicola and Antonio Ferretti

Institute of Advanced Biomedical Technologies, University of Chieti "G. D'Annunzio" and National Institute for the Physics of Matter, Research Unit of L'Aquila, Italy

Armando Tartaro and Lorenzo Bonomo

Department of Clinical Sciences and Bio-images and Institute of Advanced Biomedical Technologies, University of Chieti "G. D'Annunzio", Italy

Gian Luca Romani

Department of Clinical Sciences and Bio-images and Institute of Advanced Biomedical Technologies, University of Chieti "G. D'Annunzio", and National Institute for the Physics of Matter, Research Unit of L'Aquila, Italy

Correspondence should be addressed to Rosalia Di Matteo, Department of Clinical Sciences and Bio-images, University of Chieti "G. D'Annunzio", Via dei Vestini, 33, 66013 Chieti, Italy. Email: rosalia.dimatteo@unich.it

We would like to thank Alexander Dale for the careful reading of our paper and his helpful comments.

© 2004 Psychology Press Ltd
http://www.tandf.co.uk/journals/pp/09541446.html   DOI: 10.1080/09541440340000493

Although both imagery and perception may be related to more than one sensory input, and information coming from different sensory channels is often integrated in a unique mental representation, most recent neuroimaging literature has focused on visual imaging. Contrasting results have been obtained concerning the sharing of the same mechanisms by visual perception and visual imagery, in part due to assessment techniques and to interindividual variability in brain activation. In recent years, an increasing number of researchers have adopted novel neuroimaging techniques in order to investigate intermodal connections in mental imagery and have reported a high degree of interaction between mental imagery and other cognitive functions. In the present study the specific nature of mental imagery was investigated by means of fMRI on a more extensive set of perceptual experiences (shapes, sounds, touches, odours, flavours, self-perceived movements, and internal sensations). Results show that the left middle-inferior temporal area is recruited by mental imagery for all modalities investigated and not only for the visual one, while parietal and prefrontal areas exhibit a more heterogeneous pattern of activation across modalities. The prominent left lateralisation observed for almost all the conditions suggests that verbal cues affect the processes underlying the generation of images.

Functional neuroimaging techniques were recently supposed to contribute to settling the imagery debate about the specificity and the format of imaged representations (Farah, 2000). The question most often addressed is the sharing of mechanisms in imagery and like-modality perception (cf. Craver-Lemley, Arterberry, & Reeves, 1999; Miyashita, 1995), sometimes focusing on behavioural phenomena, brain-damaged patients (Bartolomeo et al., 1998; Levine, Warach, & Farah, 1985), and brain activation areas in imagery and perception (Kosslyn & Thompson, 2000).

Although both imagery and perception may be related to more than one sensory input, and information coming from different sensory channels is often integrated in a unique mental representation, most recent neuroimaging literature has focused on visual images. In these studies, visual imagery is usually compared with perceiving the names of concrete and/or abstract objects. These objects are presented to the subjects either visually (Kosslyn & Rabin, 1999) or aurally (D'Esposito et al., 1997; Klein, Paradis, Poline, Kosslyn, & Le Bihan, 2000; Mellet, Tzourio-Mazoyer, Denis, & Mazoyer, 1998b), or simply by matching imagery and concurrent perception (Ishai, Ungerleider, & Haxby, 2000).

The first question, that is whether visual perception and imagery share the same mechanisms, has been investigated by comparing response patterns to perceived and imaged stimuli. Some studies support the model that imagery operates in a way similar to perception by reporting perceptual and imagery impairments following posterior focal brain damage (see Kosslyn, 1994, for a review). Other studies note the activation of early stage visual processing areas during visual imagery (Chen, Kato, Zhu, Ogawa, Tank, & Ugurbil, 1998; Cohen et al., 1996; Kosslyn, Thompson, Kim, & Alpert, 1995). On the other hand, clinical studies on patients exhibiting dissociation between perceptual recognition and visual imagery seem to indicate that, in some cases, perception and imagery operate in different ways (Bartolomeo et al., 1998).

Recently, Klein et al. (2000) reported strong evidence that visual-mental imagery recruits the earliest stages of the visual system. This evidence was obtained with event-related fMRI responses to aurally presented stimuli, with both concrete and abstract characteristics of animals being imaged. However, as the authors admitted, these kinds of results are far from conclusive, in part due to the technique and the interindividual variability in the brain activation of participants, as well as to the intervening effects of attention and short-term memory.

A composite interpretation was proposed by Craver-Lemley et al. (1999). They suggested that perception and imagery might share a complementary mechanism at a low-level of processing, acting as a constraint at higher levels of processing. According to this hypothesis, perception may influence imagery at the level at which different features are conjoined because of the interference produced in the overlapping stage of object perception/image generation.

In our opinion, instead of starting by looking for a neural substrate shared by perception and imagery, we have first to define at which level of processing imagery may be constrained by perceptual factors. Kosslyn (1994) revised the model he put forward in the first part of *Image and Brain* by adding a subsystem devoted to visual image activation, and independent from immediate sensory input, to define this level of processing that involves perceptual factors.

Although several studies show that the primary visual cortex is involved in visual imagery (see above), recent evidence reveals a more complex picture when the contribution of early visual processing stages in mental imagery is excluded (D'Esposito et al., 1997). This latter position could well match the perceptual activity theories considering imagery as "a continual process of active interrogation of the environment" (Thomas, 1999, p. 218).

The interaction between long-term retrieval and control processes (attention and working memory) in mental imagery has not been adequately considered in fMRI analyses. Bruyer and Scailquin (1998) used a selective interference paradigm to test the role of specific working memory components in different visual imagery tasks. They showed that articulatory suppression, generally, does not impair imagery abilities, spatial suppression destroys image generation and image maintenance but does not impair mental transformation, and, finally, random item production affects image generation and mental transformation but leaves image maintenance unaffected. Yamamoto and Mukai (1998) found an early left lateralisation of the ERPs during an imagery task that they attributed to spatial working memory processes elicited by prefrontal areas. In their PET study Mellet et al. (1998b) found the activation of the prefrontal cortex that they attributed to the generation and transformation of mental images by working memory. However, as indicated by Braver (2001), the literature is mixed as to whether the prefrontal cortex should be considered as a storage or control component. This author hypothesises that the prefrontal cortex represents and actively maintains contextual information, which integrates storage and control functions.

The interesting attempt to clarify the format question that both Farah (2000) and Kosslyn and Thompson (2000) draw from the newest literature may be directly tied to vision as well. This is true also for the comparison between perception of visual attributes of motion and imagery tasks of similar motion in Barnes et al. (2000), or during execution and internal simulation of memorised saccadic eye movements in Höllinger, Beisteiner, Lang, Lindinger, and Berthoz (1999).

The older behavioural research may be closer to today's interest of cognitive science in sensory integration and intermodal differences among processes generated from different sensory channels. The first quantitative instrument (Betts, 1909; revised by Sheehan, 1967; White, Ashton, & Brown, 1977) was devised to evaluate mental imagery, not only in the visual modality, but also in the auditory, haptic, olfactory, gustatory, kinaesthesic, and organic ones. In particular, some of these studies investigated the relationships between visual and auditory imagery (Gissurarson, 1992), visual and kinaesthesic imagery (Farthing, Venturino, & Brown, 1983), visual imagery and olfactory stimulation (Gilbert, Crouch, & Kemp, 1998; Wolpin & Weinstein, 1983). Moreover, the investigation into the assessment of the reported vividness of experienced imagery devoted some attention to intermodal comparison (Campos & Perez, 1988; Chara, 1992; Hishitani & Murakami, 1992; Isaac, Marks, & Russell, 1986; Marks, 1989; Marks & Isaac, 1995).

In recent years, an increasing number of researchers adopted novel neuro-imaging techniques in order to investigate intermodal connections (see for example, Fallgatter, Mueller, & Strik, 1997; Farah, Weisberg, Monheit, & Peronnet, 1990). However, due to differences in techniques and methodology, it is often not easy to put together results concerning imagery modalities, although, as Mellet, Petit, Mazoyer, Denis, and Tzourio-Mazoyer (1998a) pointed out, these studies indicate a high degree of interaction between mental imagery and other cognitive functions.

Consequently, we decided to investigate the specific nature of mental imagery by studying the imagery process on a more extensive set of perceptual experiences, using an fMRI analysis. The present study involved an fMRI block recording during which participants were requested to generate mental images cued by short sentences describing different perceptual experiences (shapes, sounds, touches, odours, flavours, self-perceived movements, and internal sensations). Imagery cues were presented in written form and were contrasted with sentences describing abstract concepts, since differences in activation during visual imagery and abstract thoughts were often assessed in the literature (Goldenberg, Podreka, Steiner, & Willmes, 1987; Lehman, Kochi, Koenig,

Koykkou, Michel, & Strik, 1994; Petsche, Lacroix, Lindner, Rappelsberger, & Schmidt, 1992; Wise et al., 2000).

METHOD

Participants

Fifteen healthy volunteers, after signing an informed consent waiver, participated in this study. The study was approved by the university ethics committee. Six participants were female and nine were male. All ranged between 18 and 20 in age. Participants were paid about €25 for their participation in this study. Handedness was assessed by asking a set of simple questions regarding the performance of everyday acts. Participants were enrolled in the study only if (1) they were right handed according to this test, and (2) reported that both their parents were right handed as well.

Design

The experimental task required subjects to generate mental images cued by visually presented written stimuli. Each experimental session of a single subject consisted of three fMRI runs and a morphological MRI.

In each run, three stimuli from one experimental condition (regarding one of the seven selected modalities) were alternated with three stimuli from the control condition three times. Overall, nine different experimental stimuli and nine different control stimuli were presented in each run.

The experimental stimuli in one of the three runs always belonged to the visual modality, while those in the other two runs were evenly divided among the remaining six modalities. The visual modality was always included in each experimental session and used as a reference. In this way, the visual modality was studied fifteen times, while each of the other six modalities was studied five times. The number of modalities studied for each subject was limited to three in order to avoid lengthy recording sessions. The fifteen subjects may therefore be grouped by modality, yielding three groups of five subjects: (1) the "auditory-olfactory" group, (2) the "tactile-gustatory" group, and (3) the "kinaesthesic-organic" group.

Each run was performed according to a block paradigm, in which functional image acquisitions (volumes) during mental imagery, i.e., during experimental stimulus delivery—were alternated with functional image acquisitions during baseline, i.e., during control sentence delivery. Precisely, a block of 12 volumes during mental imagery was followed by a block of 12 volumes during the control condition, and this sequence was repeated three times, for 72 volumes. Experimental and control stimuli were presented at the start of the first, and then of every fourth volume, so that three different experimental stimuli or three different control stimuli, were presented in each block. Each stimulus, or control sentence, remained visible until it was replaced by the following. Thus, subjects could see every stimulus for the whole time interval corresponding to the acquisition of four volumes, i.e., 24 s. The duration of a block was therefore 72 s, and the total duration of a run was 7 min 12 s.

Stimulus material

The stimulus material consisted of eight sets of sentences referring to either concrete or abstract objects. Seven sets were used in the experimental condition and the remaining one was used in the control condition as baseline. Each experimental set consisted of nine sentences, whereas the control set consisted of 27 sentences, and each sentence was composed of three or four words.

The experimental sets contained sentences identifying a definite perceptual experience and referring respectively to the visual, auditory, tactile, olfactory, gustatory, kinaesthesic, and organic modalities. The control set contained sentences referring to abstract concepts.

An English translation of a sentence exemplar in each set is: *seeing a coin* (visual), *hearing a rumble* (auditory), *touching a soft material* (tactile), *smelling wet paint* (olfactory), *tasting a salty food* (gustatory), *the act of walking* (kinaesthesic), *feeling tired* (organic), *admitting a misdeed* (abstract).

The correspondence between the experimenters' classification of the sentences and the corresponding mental images was tested in a preliminary behavioural study, in which 57 first-year university students rated the entire set of stimuli. None of them participated in the fMRI study.

The behavioural study required participants to classify each sentence according to the most prominent imagery modality (multiple choice response) and to rate the vividness of the image evoked by the corresponding sentence (scale range of 1–7). The data from the behavioural study were particularly important concerning the abstract items as these items were included in the sentence sets in order to form the baseline condition against which to evaluate the modality specific conditions.

Chi-square comparison for each modality between observed and expected frequencies revealed that participants' responses significantly matched the item classification, $p < .001$. Moreover, the rating of the power to evoke mental images (image vividness) revealed that modality specific items obtained an average rating of 4.85 ($SD = 1.09$), while abstract items only achieved an average value of 2.97 ($SD = 1.05$), $t = 6.17$, $p < .0001$. The result was confirmed also for each single modality vs. abstract items comparison, $p < .001$ for each comparison.

The entire set of stimuli was presented for rating also to the participants of the present study, after the end of the fMRI session in which only the stimuli of three modalities were presented to each subject. In this case, chi-square comparisons showed again that participants' responses significantly matched the item classification, $p < .001$, and vividness ratings of modality specific items (mean 5.30, $SD = 1.03$) were significantly higher, $t = 11.98$, $p < .0001$, than those of abstract items (mean 2.10, $SD = 1.22$). The difference was confirmed also for each of the single comparisons, $p < .001$. Data on both ratings are summarised in Table 1. Although the results obtained in the preliminary study are slightly different from those obtained from the participants in the fMRI study, they roughly correspond to one another.

Some explanation is needed for the two sentence sets that obtained a rather low rate particularly by the fMRI group. In the case of abstract items rated as no images, the low rate is mainly due to the fact that some participants judged most of them as evoking an image related to an internal sensation (organic image). As these images do not seem consistently related to other modalities, the abstract items were judged suitable to serve as baseline condition in the fMRI study.

Conversely, the organic images' low rate seems due to the dispersion of the organic items across different sensory modalities, while the minor rate of the kinaesthesic items in fMRI group seemed to be related to major rate of classification in the visual category. Although the organic and kinaesthesic items seemed to evoke images in other modalities as well, it should be noted that no modality was directly compared to another one in the fMRI study (each modality was evaluated against the abstract baseline condition).

For image vividness, in both the preliminary study and the subsequent one with the fMRI group, the mean vividness ratings for abstract items were significantly lower than those for modality-specific items, that did not differ among them. This difference represents a further confirmation of the validity of using the abstract set as a baseline condition against which all other modalities stimuli are evaluated.

Procedure

Participants were acquainted with the experimental apparatus and were interviewed in order to verify the lack of contraindications of participating in the experiment. They were informed they would be presented with a set of sentences and were instructed to mentally read them, without moving their lips, to concentrate on them, and try to imagine their content.

Experimental and control sentences were projected on a translucent glass placed on the back of the scanner bore by means of an LCD projector and two perpendicular mirrors. An additional mirror fixed to the head coil inside the magnet bore allowed the subject to see the translucent glass. The LCD projector was driven by a PC placed at the scanner console and connected to it via a VGA cable through a hole in the shielded room. Event timing was manually controlled by the PC operator. The stimuli and control sentences were administered by means of slide presentation software, and were printed in yellow on a blue background. No artifacts due to either the projector or the VGA cable were visible in the functional as well as in the morphological images.

TABLE 1

The table shows the proportions of item classification according to each multiple-choice category and vividness ratings for the preliminary study and the fMRI study

Items	Multiple-choice categories								Vividness ratings	
	Visual	Auditory	Tactile	Olfactory	Gustatory	Kinaesthesic	Organic	None	Mean	SD
Preliminary study (57 cases)										
visual	**0.93**	0.01	0.02	0.01	0.00	0.01	0.01	0.02	5.50	0.98
auditory	0.05	**0.89**	0.00	0.00	0.00	0.02	0.01	0.02	4.75	1.06
tactile	0.03	0.00	**0.89**	0.00	0.02	0.01	0.04	0.02	4.86	1.05
olfactory	0.01	0.01	0.00	**0.94**	0.01	0.00	0.01	0.01	4.66	1.06
gustatory	0.01	0.00	0.00	0.03	**0.93**	0.00	0.03	0.02	4.72	1.03
kinaesthesic	0.07	0.00	0.03	0.01	0.00	**0.84**	0.03	0.02	4.71	1.24
organic	0.02	0.01	0.09	0.01	0.11	0.08	**0.59**	0.10	4.61	1.13
abstract	0.07	0.04	0.00	0.00	0.00	0.03	0.23	**0.63**	2.97	1.05
fMRI study (15 cases)										
visual	**0.96**	0.00	0.01	0.00	0.00	0.00	0.01	0.01	6.10	0.78
auditory	0.13	**0.85**	0.00	0.00	0.00	0.00	0.00	0.02	5.18	0.96
tactile	0.07	0.00	**0.88**	0.00	0.02	0.00	0.03	0.00	5.14	0.96
olfactory	0.04	0.01	0.00	**0.90**	0.00	0.00	0.00	0.03	5.00	1.05
gustatory	0.06	0.00	0.00	0.01	**0.89**	0.01	0.00	0.03	4.81	1.15
kinaesthesic	0.19	0.00	0.03	0.00	0.00	**0.74**	0.00	0.02	5.81	0.86
organic	0.08	0.01	0.10	0.00	0.11	0.10	**0.47**	0.12	4.95	1.10
abstract	0.09	0.05	0.00	0.00	0.00	0.04	0.28	**0.55**	2.10	1.22

Apparatus

Functional MRI was performed with a Siemens Vision 1.5T scanner with EPI (Echo Planar Imaging) capability. Each functional volume was acquired by means of an EPI FID (Free Induction Decay) sequence with the following parameters: 30 bicommisural transaxial slices 3 mm thickness, no gap, matrix 64 × 64, FOV (Field Of View) 192, 3 mm × 3 mm in-plane voxel size, flip angle 90°, TR 6 s, TE 60 ms. That image covered the whole brain.

In addition to functional images, a high resolution, morphological MRI was acquired at the end of each session, by means of a 3D-MPRAGE (Magnetisation Prepared Rapid Gradient Echo) sequence. The parameters characterising this acquisition were: 240 axial slices, 1 mm thickness, no gap, matrix 256 × 256, FOV 256 mm, in-plane voxel size 1 mm × 1 mm, flip angle 12°, TR = 9.7 ms, TE = 4 ms.

Data analysis

Individual analysis.   Functional data were analysed using MEDx software by Sensor Systems. First, all volumes in a run were realigned, in order to correct for physiological subject movement. All functional volumes were transformed into Talairach space. The volumes were grouped by modality, and, in each modality were further divided into subgroups corresponding to volumes acquired during the presentation of modality specific stimuli, and during the presentation of control sentences respectively. Voxel time courses were high pass filtered with a time constant of 288 seconds, corresponding to the duration of two pairs of blocks of volumes. Then data for each subject and sensory modality were analysed according to the General Linear Model, and the corresponding Z-score maps were calculated and thresholded at $Z = 2.3$ corresponding to a null probability $p < .01$ (uncorrected). Subsequently, activation was selected by means of a clustering algorithm keeping only the clusters of activation with a size equal to, or larger than 5 voxels. This corresponded to a rate of false positive of 5% as calculated by means of a simulation, taking into account the image matrix and Z-score level (Cox, 1996). Clusters were then classified, for each subject and modality, according to their neuroanatomical location, by means of the Talairach atlas.

Group analysis.   In addition, in order to increase the signal to noise ratio, a group analysis was performed for each sensory modality, by calculating a group Z-score map from the individual Z-score maps of individual subjects in that modality. This procedure consisted in a normalised average of all Z-score maps. The individual nonclustered Z-score maps were used, and the resulting group Z-score map was thresholded at $Z = 2.3$ and clustered afterwards, at the same statistical significance level as in the individual study (5%).

RESULTS

The pattern of activation derived from the group analysis for each modality is summarised in Table 2 and will be presented before the individual analyses.

In the visual modality, the most prominent areas of activation were observed, bilaterally, in the inferior parietal lobule, in the middle temporal gyrus and in the inferior temporal gyrus. Another prominent activation was observed in the right middle-inferior frontal areas, while only a small activation was found in the right middle frontal areas (see Figure 1a).

TABLE 2
Talairach coordinates for the activated areas in the different modalities

Area	Visual Left x, y, z	Visual Right x, y, z	Auditory Left x, y, z	Auditory Right x, y, z	Tactile Left x, y, z	Tactile Right x, y, z
Fusiform/hippocampal gyrus (BA37)	−33, 39, −19					
Inferior temporal gyrus (BA37)	−61, −64, −9	57, −57, −7	−66, −60, −4		−50, −5, −4	
Middle temporal gyrus (BA22/37)	−57, −62, 5	48, −60, 7	−58, 2, 0			
Insula		38, −14, −4	−43, −1, −14			
Precuneus (BA7)	−23, −72, 57	28, −64, 57				
Superior parietal lobule (BA7)						
Inferior parietal lobule (BA40)	−59, −29, 47	59, −37, 41	−61, −35, 41		−63, −32, 41	
Medial frontal gyrus (BA6)						
Superior frontal gyrus (BA6)						
Middle frontal gyrus (BA6)		30, 1, 64			−24, −11, 57	
Middle frontal gyrus (BA9/10)	−36, 42, 44	42, 42, 25				
Middle-inferior frontal gyrus (BA44/46)		47, 21, 28	−50, 36, 17	49, 16, 24	−59, 11, 28	60, 15, 25
Middle frontal gyrus (BA11)	−32, 37, −20	31, 39, −18				

In the auditory modality, the main areas of activation were, bilaterally, in the middle-inferior frontal gyrus (more intense on the left) and in the left middle and inferior temporal areas (see Figure 1b). Activated areas were found also in the left inferior parietal lobule. The left hemisphere seems to be more activated than the right one.

Figure 1c shows the activation pattern for the tactile modality. It is quite asymmetrical, with most prominent activation in the left hemisphere, where activated areas were observed in the inferior temporal gyrus and in the inferior

TABLE 2
(Continued)

Modality and hemispheres							
Olfactory		Gustatory		Kinaesthesic		Organic	
Left x, y, z	Right x, y, z	Left x, y, z	Right x, y, z	Left x, y, z	Right x, y, z	Left x, y, z	Right x, y, z
		−52, −57, −16					
		−47, −4, −6		−61, −58, −3	50, −61, 4		
−64, 0, 9						−64, −5, 6	
−42, −1, 5			40, 7, −10				
−15, −72, 48			13, −69, 34				
				−23, −52, 68			
−64, −25, 33	64, −25, 33	−61, −35, 43	49, −37, 57	−58, −32, 47	54, −28, 48	−63, −29, 49	54, −26, 53
		−3, −16, 57		−5, −9, 58			
				−24, −1, 63	25, −8, 66		
−49, 37, 13	38, 38, 12	−53, 41, 6	44, 44, 4				
			26, 34, −15				

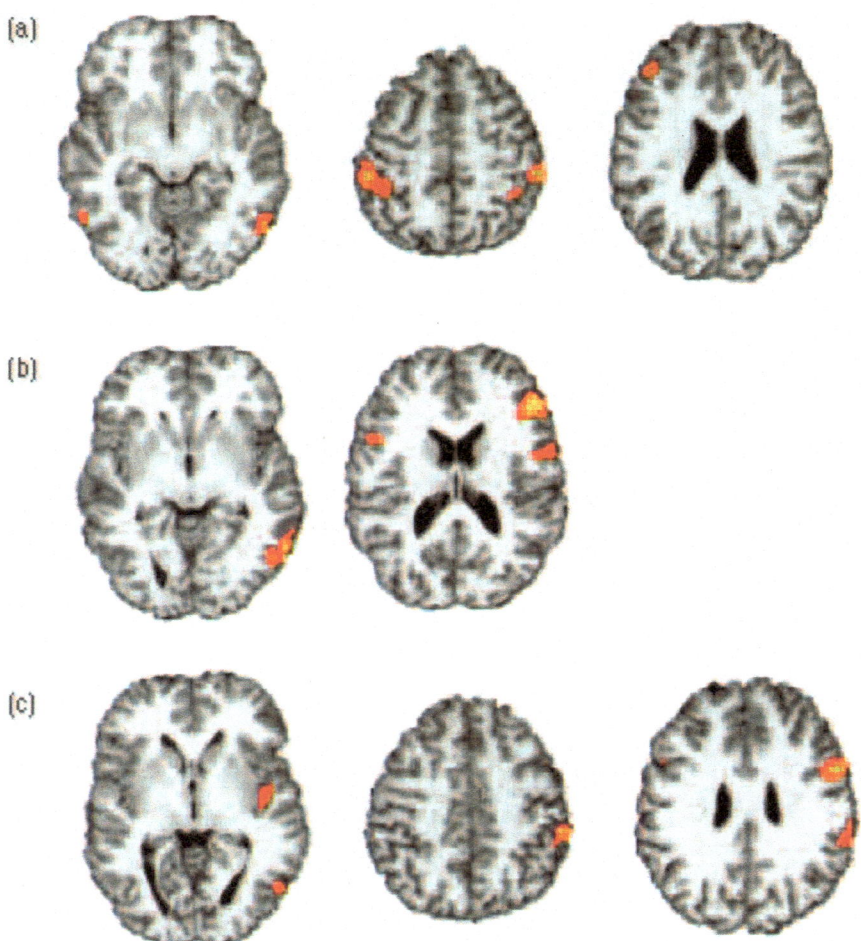

Figure 1. The figure shows active areas for: **(a)** visual modality, bilaterally, in the middle-inferior temporal cortex (left panel), and in the inferior parietal lobule (central panel) and on the right hemisphere in the middle frontal area (right panel), **(b)** auditory modality in the left middle-inferior temporal cortex (left panel) and, bilaterally, in the middle-inferior frontal cortex (right panel), **(c)** tactile modality mainly on the left hemisphere in the inferior temporal cortex (left panel), in the inferior parietal lobule (central and right panel) and in the middle-inferior frontal cortex (right panel).

parietal lobule. A bilateral activation was found in the inferior frontal gyrus (see Table 2).

In the olfactory condition, bilateral areas of activation were observed in the inferior parietal lobule and in the middle frontal gyrus (more intense on the left). In the left hemisphere, predominant activations were observed in the middle temporal gyrus (see Figure 2a).

For the gustatory modality, activated areas in both hemispheres were in the inferior parietal lobule, and in the middle frontal gyrus. In the left hemisphere, areas of activation were observed in the hippocampal fusiform gyrus and in the inferior temporal cortex (see Figure 2b). A large activated area was found in the right insula with no symmetric counterpart and in the left medial frontal cortex.

For the kinaesthesic modality, Figure 2c shows a rather symmetrical activation in the inferior parietal lobule, and in the middle-inferior temporal gyrus. In the left hemisphere, activation was observed in the superior parietal lobule. A left-centred activation was observed also in the medial frontal area.

The organic modality showed a bilateral compound symmetrical activation pattern around the inferior parietal lobule (see Figure 2d).

Data from individual analyses were grouped according to three different regions and statistical comparisons across modalities[1] on the number of activated voxels in each condition and hemisphere were performed separately within each group of subjects.[2] These regions were the middle-inferior temporal cortex (BA37 and 22), the lateral parietal cortex (BA39 and 40), and the lateral prefrontal cortex (BA9, 10, 44, 45, 46), and were chosen among those areas that were found to be more active in a preliminary analysis,[3] in order to examine in detail the corresponding pattern of activation. As we will see, results from the two types of analysis are not perfectly coincident, because part of the individually activated clusters are lost in the group analysis due to both slight spatial disparities and differences in cluster's extent among individual patterns of activation.

For the middle-inferior temporal cortex, the 3×2 ANOVAs (Modality $\times$ Hemisphere) carried out separately for each group on the number of activated voxels reveal a greater activation on the left hemisphere for the visual, auditory, tactile, olfactory, and gustatory modalities, $F(1, 4) = 21.707, p < .01; F(1, 4) = 110.645, p < .001$. The kinaesthesic and the organic modalities did not show any significant difference between the left and the right side.

---

[1] The comparison between the visual modality and the other ones in terms of overlapping activation was discussed in Olivetti Belardinelli, Di Matteo, Del Gratta, De Nicola, Ferretti, and Romani (2004).

[2] Preliminarily, in order to assess rough differences in the pattern of activation among the three groups of subjects in the visual modality (see the Design section), a 3×2 ANOVA (Group $\times$ Hemisphere) was carried out on the number of activated voxels for each participant in the visual condition. Results did not indicate the existence of significant differences, thus allowing a consistent comparison, within each group of subjects, of other sensory modalities with the visual one.

[3] The preliminary analysis was presented as the Eighth European Workshop on Imagery and Cognition, Saint-Malo, France, April 1–3, 2001.

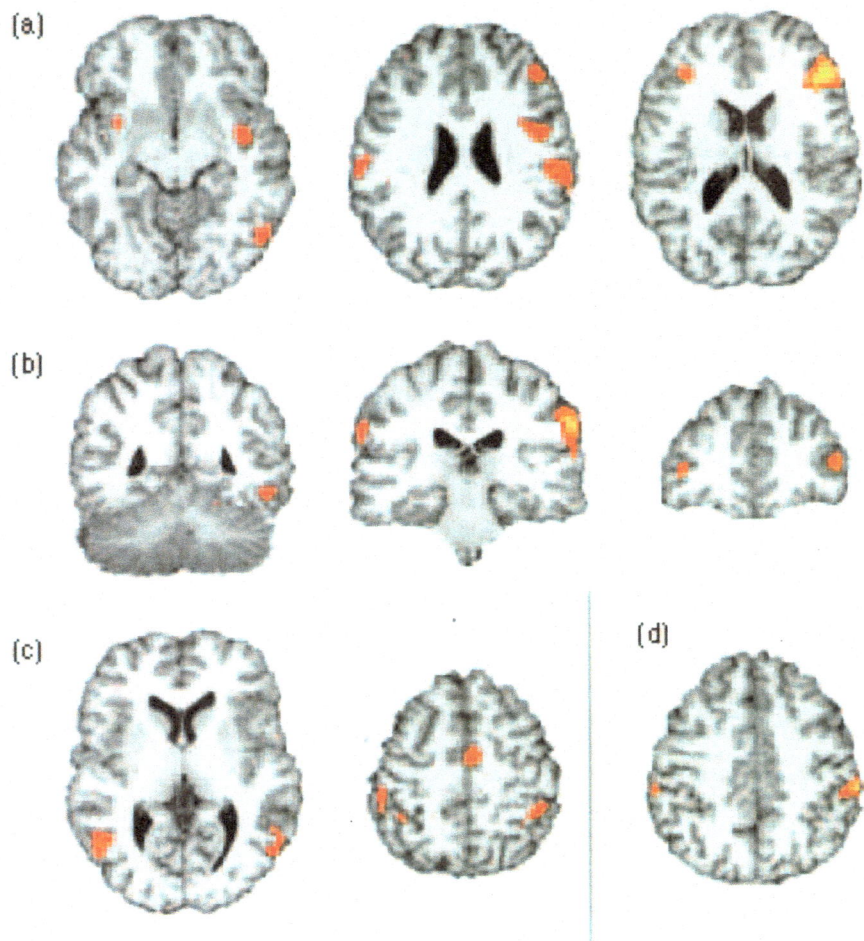

Figure 2. The figure shows active areas for: **(a)** olfactory modality in the left middle temporal cortex (left panel), in the insula (left and central panel), in the parietal cortex (central panel) and in the middle frontal cortex (right panel), **(b)** gustatory modality in the left inferior temporal cortex and in the fusiform gyrus (left panel), and bilaterally in the parietal cortex (central panel) and in the middle frontal cortex (right panel), **(c)** kinaesthesic modality, bilaterally, in the inferior temporal cortex (left panel) and in the parietal cortex (centre). The activation of the medial frontal cortex is also shown (central panel), **(d)** organic modality in the parietal cortex of both hemispheres (right panel).

742

The 3 × 2 ANOVAs (Modality × Hemisphere) on the number of activated voxels in the lateral intermodal analysis of mental imagery parietal cortex showed a Modality × Hemisphere interaction, $F(2, 8) = 5.092$, $p < .05$; LSD test with $p < .05$. The significance of the effect comes from the tactile condition having a greater activation on the left hemisphere than on the right. The other modalities did not show any significant difference among activated areas.

The 3 × 2 ANOVAs (Modality × Hemisphere) for the lateral prefrontal cortex also showed a Modality × Hemisphere interaction, $F(2, 8) = 7.002$, $p < .02$. In this case, the effect is that the activation of the visual modality was greater on the right than on the left, while the activation of the olfactory modality shows the opposite pattern with the activation on the left greater than the activation on the right. Moreover, on the left hemisphere the activation for the auditory and the olfactory modalities was greater than the activation for the visual modality (LSD test with $p < .05$). The other two groups did not show any significant differences.

DISCUSSION

Our study shows that the generation of mental images from different sensory modalities is associated with a composite pattern of brain activation that involves functional circuits which vary with the modality.

Firstly, the present data show that mental images activate regions of the posterior temporal cortex in both hemispheres. This activation was significantly more pronounced on the left hemisphere for almost all modalities, and it was independent from the sensory modality supposed to elicit the images.

Secondly, bilateral activation was observed in the parietal cortex for almost all the modalities, although the volume of activation was significantly larger for the tactile modality, particularly in the left hemisphere.

Finally, bilateral activation in several regions of the prefrontal cortex was also found, with larger activation for the olfactory modality in the left hemisphere and for the visual modality in the right hemisphere.

Primary areas were not found to be very active and, although no direct comparisons were made between perceptual and imagery processes in different sensory modalities, this circumstance suggests that different interactive neural circuits underlie low- and high-level processes.

In considering the specific pattern of activation related to each modality, our data on visual imagery seems to be consistent with the data reported in the literature (Cocude, Mellet, & Denis, 1999; D'Esposito et al., 1997; De Volder et al., 2001; Mellet et al., 1998b; Mellet et al., 2000). However, since we found only occasional clusters of activation in the occipital lobe, the present study is at odds with others reporting activation in primary visual area (Chen et al., 1998; Klein et al., 2000; Kosslyn & Thompson, 2000). The lack of any consistent activation of primary visual areas could be due to the kind of task used in this study. As suggested by Thompson, Kosslyn, Sukel, and Alpert (2001), primary visual cortex is activated more often when participants are requested to use the image in some way. In our study, in order to minimise differences among the conditions, apart from those related to the imagery modality, participants were simply requested to mentally represent the target item, i.e., they were requested to perform an image generation task. According to Behrmann (2000), image generation is a process more specific to imagery than image manipulation, because it involves the active reconstruction of a long-term mental representation. Moreover, in our opinion, image manipulation involves some kinds of online processing that might be more dependent on the specific content of the image to be manipulated. An alternative explanation for the lack of activation of primary visual areas may be due to the visual presentation of the imagery cues that may have cancelled the specific visual processing components. However, studies that contrasted concrete items vs. abstract items by using an auditory presentation instead of a visual one (D'Esposito et al., 1997; De Volder et al., 2001; Mellet et al., 1998b) found substantially the same pattern of results.

Regarding the auditory modality, we observed predominantly left activation on the inferior temporal lobe and in the parietal cortex and a bilateral activation in the prefrontal cortex. This result contrasts with other data. Zatorre and Halpern (1993) reported that the right temporal lobectomy causes impairments in both perception and imagery for songs, while the left one leaves performance on both tasks relatively unaffected. Zatorre, Halpern, Perry, Meyer, and Evans (1996) compared the PET data from auditory perception of songs to those derived from corresponding auditory imagery and found that the same brain regions were activated in the two tasks, that is the secondary auditory cortex, and areas in the prefrontal and parietal lobes. However, in both studies, the stimuli to be imaged are songs, while our stimuli are typical sounds from highly familiar objects. It is possible that processing of pitch and melody involves different neural regions and cognitive processes.

Tactile imagery exhibits predominantly left activation in the posterior cerebral area (temporal and parietal) and bilateral activation in prefrontal areas. Our data are in line with event-related potentials data on visual, auditory, and tactile imagery reported by Fallgatter et al. (1997), showing a left posterior lateralisation of the P300 centroid in the tactile imagery condition, as opposed to a right lateralisation in the visual imagery condition, and a midline localisation in the auditory imagery condition. According to the authors, these asymmetries may reflect the simultaneous activity of distributed modality specific cortical areas. The left hemisphere predominance for the tactile modality was reported also by Findlay, Ashton, and McFarland (1994), by showing faster response at generating images from categorically stored information as opposed to globally stored information. Although, it is not possible to exclude

that these asymmetries may be related to the right-handedness of the participants, a prominent left activation is observed also for the olfactory and gustatory modalities. This left activation can hardly be explained by means of
subjects' right-handedness.

In fact, although the olfactory and gustatory modalities show distributed
bilateral activation, they exhibit a more intense involvement of the left hemisphere mainly in the temporal and (only for the olfactory) in the prefrontal areas.
For the olfactory modality, Savic (2001) reported that different memory tasks on
odours are mediated by common, as well as task-specific, regions into the limbic
cortex (piriform, orbito-frontal, cingulate, insular cortices). Moreover, it is
known that the gustatory system too exhibits strong connections with limbic
structures, as was further documented by Spector (2000) in a recent review.
Nevertheless, we did not find any evidence of conspicuous activation of limbic
structures. However, the mainly left lateralisation of the patterns of activation
we observed is coherent with the indication reported by Kosslyn et al. (1993),
suggesting that the left hemisphere generates images by using categorial spatial
description whereas the right hemisphere generates images by using precise
spatial references. In fact, taste, smell and touch may be represented without a
direct reference to an external space organisation, whereas visual, auditory,
kinaesthesic, and organic representation rely on a space reference system. This
interpretation is in line with the distinction between a nonspatial and a spatial
relational encoding put forward by Rugg (1997) while reviewing data on
olfaction memory.

Since kinaesthesic imagery requires the internal rehearsal of simple or
complex motor acts without accompaniment of overt movements, it may be
preferentially defined motor imagery. Although motor/kinaesthesic imagery
presents some similarities with mental manipulation tasks, a distinction must be
drawn between the two types of imagery. In the attempt to differentiate motor
images from other types of images (e.g., visual), Jeannerod (1995) described
motor images as the result of the "first person" process involving mostly a
kinaesthesic representation of the action, implying that subjects feel themselves
executing a given action. According to the author, motor/kinaesthesic imagery
requires a representation of the body as the generator of acting forces and not
only of the effects of these forces on the external world. By consequence, the
central question in the studies on this topic is whether motor images share the
same neural mechanisms that are also responsible for the preparation of actual
movements (Mellet et al., 1998a). In fact, several studies that compared overt
and imagined movements by means of psycho-physiological and neuroimaging
techniques, found activation either in the Supplementary Motor Area (Höllinger
et al., 1999; Rao et al., 1993; Stephan et al., 1995), or in the primary motor
cortex (Bodis-Wollner, Bucher, Seelos, Paulus, Reiser, & Oertel, 1997; Porro et
al., 1996; Roth et al., 1996). In the present case, we did not find any evidence of
the involvement of these areas in our kinaesthesic condition. This may be

because in our study imaged movements according to the presented stimuli referred to several different complex actions and did not regard simple and repetitive movements often used in other studies. These circumstances introduce inevitable differences in our study that do not permit a direct comparison with the previous ones.

Finally, the organic modality shows a less definite pattern of activation than other modalities even if it involves the temporal and parietal cortex as the other modalities do. This could be due to the use of a less definite imagery cue in the experimental procedure as we saw from the separate item classifications (see Table 1). However, we may observe that the pattern of activation that accompanies the organic modality was confined to the posterior cerebral cortex in a greater measure than other modalities; and these results seem to support the idea of an amodal neuronal circuit sustaining high-level imagery processes.

In all modalities, activation of the posterior portion of the middle-inferior temporal cortex was observed. Although several studies reported the activation of this area in visual imagery, some of them (Farah, 1995; Iwaki, Ueno, Imada, & Tonoike, 1999) show a left-sided focus, while others present either no asymmetry or a right lateralisation (Kosslyn et al., 1993). In particular, Farah (1995), reviewing data on brain damage and neuroimaging studies, concluded that the left hemisphere appears to be specialised in image generation, although both hemispheres are presumably involved. D'Esposito et al. (1997) also found a left activation of this area in the majority of their subjects, by using an image generation task cued by concrete and abstract words. Nevertheless, Mellet et al. (1998a) suggested that the analysis of shapes accounts for the right hemisphere activation, whereas the verbal transformation accounts for the left hemisphere activation. From their point of view, the different experimental result depends on obstacles either to perform a detailed analysis of the shapes (for example, by generating an image every 1 s, as in D'Esposito et al., 1997), or to verbalise the generated images (for example by using complex shapes, as in Mellet, Tzourio-Mazoyer, Crivello, Joliot, Denis, & Mazoyer, 1996).

Our results confirm the relevance of the inferior temporal area in visual imagery and extend its role to other sensory modalities. In fact, we found the posterior middle-inferior temporal region activated bilaterally in almost all the modalities even if the left-side activation was often more pronounced. This area receives information derived from different sensory modalities (e.g., visual, auditory, somatosensory). Moreover, it is linked with both the ventral system of object recognition (Stewart, Meyer, Frith, & Rothwell, 2001; Thompson-Schill, Aguirre, D'Esposito, & Farah, 1999) and the dorsolateral system involved in visuospatial processing (Cocude et al., 1999; Haxby, Hoewitz, Ungerleider, Maisog, Pietrini, & Grady, 1994). Wise et al. (2000) suggested that the left side of this area may have a role in connecting the verbal encoding of a word with its deeper representation, while Thompson-Schill et al. (1999) indicated that this area may reflect the segregation of semantic knowledge into anatomically discrete, but highly interactive, modality specific regions. Since in our study, all the images were cued by verbal items and each item was delivered for about 24 s, the left hemisphere predominance seems to be coherent with the hemisphere functional specialisation hypothesis.

The parietal cortex is activated bilaterally in all the modalities, even if for the tactile one a stronger activation was found on the left hemisphere. Activation in this area was also found by Barnes et al. (2000), with fMRI recorded while subjects were performing spatial mental rotations. They suggest that the inferior parietal lobule seems to be specifically recruited whenever the generation of the mental image relies on spatial processing (Banati, Goerres, Tjoa, Aggleton, & Grasby, 2000; Diwadkar, Carpenter, & Just, 2000; Iwaki et al., 1999). According to the literature, this area may be a candidate region to which modality specific information is transformed in supramodal representations. Several authors (Coull & Frith, 1998; Coull & Nobre, 1998; Jordan, Heinze, Lutz, Kanowski, & Länche, 2001) have suggested that the network underlying this transformation may be involved in low-level attentional processes, working for many types of cognitive processes. In this view, the activated areas we found in the parietal region may reflect supramodal transformations. Although it is not possible to exclude that the prominent left parietal activation in response to tactile imagery may be due to the right-handedness of the subjects, some authors have suggested a hemispheric functional specialisation for this area distinguishing a left verbal-attention processing as opposed to a right spatial-attention processing (Jordan et al., 2001).

The lateral prefrontal cortex presents a cluster of activation in both hemi-spheres for all the modalities. This area is known to be responsible for working memory operations (for a review, see Miller, 2000 and Rushworth & Owen, 1998), even though the functional organisation of the prefrontal cortex is a matter of debate. Some authors (Goldman-Rakic, 2000; Wilson, Ó Scalaidhe, & Goldman-Rakic, 1993) have hypothesised a modality or domain-specificity of the prefrontal cortex; others (Owen, Evans, & Petrides, 1996) have suggested a functional specialisation. Both these hypotheses support the idea that this region may be related to the retrieval of stored information in mental imagery. In our study, we found a composite pattern of activation distributed bilaterally, but slightly more pronounced on the left hemisphere, in particular for the olfactory modality. For what concerns the olfactory modality, in their review of neuro-imaging studies, Brand, Millot, and Henquell (2001) and Zald and Pardo (2000) reported that the perception of olfactory stimuli activates mainly the right pre-frontal cortex, while judgements on the hedonic valence of odours produce an asymmetric activation with a left-sided activation for pleasant odours. Although these data refer to a perceptual task and can supply only indirect indication to olfactory imagery, they suggested that cognitive and motivational factors may heavily affect odour processing. Regarding the other modalities, several authors (Bosch, Mecklinger, & Friederici, 2001; Burbaud, Camus, Guehl, Bioulac,

Caillé, & Allard, 2000) have reported that spatial tasks tend to activate the right prefrontal cortex, whereas verbal tasks involve mainly the left or bilateral prefrontal cortex.

We can derive some provisional conclusions. Firstly, the left middle-inferior temporal area seems to be recruited by mental imagery for all the modalities investigated in this study, and not only for the visual modality. By consequence, this area seems to be responsible either for the verbal retrieval of long-term representations or for the segregation of long-term representations into highly interactive modality specific regions.

Secondly, the pattern of activation that characterises the involvement of parietal and prefrontal areas across modalities represents further evidence for the modality-specific hypothesis advanced for the frontoparietal stream underlying working memory and attentional processes.

Thirdly, the prominent left lateralisation observed for almost all the conditions suggests that verbal cues affect the processes underlying the generation of images. Further investigations are required to better understand the nature of this influence.

In summary, the involvement of the temporoparietal and frontal circuit was observed for all the imagery modalities examined in this study. Although the specific areas activated by each modality show also a certain spatial discrepancy, the emerging picture suggests that mental image generation requires high-level processes that are largely independent from the specific representational modality.

PrEview proof published online May 2004

REFERENCES

Banati, R. B., Goerres, G. W., Tjoa, C., Aggleton, J. P., & Grasby, P. (2000). The functional anatomy of visual–tactile integration in man: A study using positron emission tomography. *Neuropsychologia, 38,* 115–124.

Barnes, J., Howard, R. J., Senior, C., Brammer, M., Bullmore, E. T., Simmons, A., Woodruff, P., & David, A. S. (2000). Cortical activity during rotational and linear transformations. *Neuropsychologia, 38,* 1148–1156.

Bartolomeo, P., Bachoud-Levi, A.-C., De Gelder, B., Denes, G., Dalla Barba, G., Brugieres, P., & Degos, J. D. (1998). Multiple-domain dissociation between impaired visual perception and preserved mental imagery in a patient with bilateral extrastriate lesions. *Neuropsychologia, 36,* 239–249.

Behrmann, M. (2000). The mind's eye mapped onto the brain's matter. *Current Directions in Psychological Science, 9,* 50–54.

Betts, G. H. (1909). *The distribution and functions of mental imagery.* New York: New York Teachers College, Columbia University.

Bodis-Wollner, I., Bucher, S. F., Seelos, K. C., Paulus, W., Reiser, M., & Oertel, W. H. (1997). Functional MRI mapping of occipital and frontal activity during voluntary and imagined saccades. *Neurology, 49,* 416–420.

Bosch, V., Mecklinger, A., & Friederici, A. D. (2001). Slow cortical potentials during retention of object, spatial, and verbal information. *Cognitive Brain Research, 10*, 219–237.

Brand, G., Millot, J.-L., & Henquell, D. (2001). Complexity of olfactory lateralization processes revealed by functional imaging: A review. *Neuroscience and Biobehavioral Reviews, 25*, 159–166.

Braver, T. S. (2001). Working memory, cognitive control and the prefrontal cortex. Computational and empirical studies. *Cognitive Processing, 2*, 25–55.

Bruyer, R., & Scailquin, J. (1998). The visuospatial sketchpad for mental images: Testing the multicomponent. *Acta Psychologica, 98*, 117–136.

Burbaud, P., Camus, O., Guehl, D., Bioulac, B., Caillé, J.-M., & Allard, M. (2000). Influence of cognitive strategies on the pattern of cortical activation during mental subtraction: A functional imaging study in human subjects. *Neuroscience Letters, 287*, 76–80.

Campos, A., & Perez, M. J. (1988). Vividness of Movement Imagery questionnaire: Relations with other measures of mental imagery. *Perceptual and Motor Skills, 67*, 607–610.

Chara, P. J., Jr. (1992). Some concluding thoughts on the debate about the Vividness of Visual Imagery Questionnaire. *Perceptual and Motor Skills, 75*, 947–954.

Chen, W., Kato, T., Zhu, X.-H., Ogawa, S., Tank, D. W., & Ugurbil, K. (1998). Human primary visual cortex and lateral geniculate nucleus activation during visual imagery. *Neuroreport, 9*, 3669–3674.

Cocude, M., Mellet, E., & Denis, M. (1999). Visual and mental exploration of visuo-spatial configurations: Behavioral and neuroimaging approaches. *Psychological Research, 62*, 93–106.

Cohen, M. S., Kosslyn, S. M., Breiter, H. C., Di Girolamo, D. J., Thompson, W. L., Anderson, A. K., Bookheimer, S. Y., Rosen, B. R., & Belliveau, J. W. (1996). Changes in cortical activity during mental rotation: A mapping study using functional magnetic resonance imaging. *Brain, 119*, 89–100.

Coull, J. T., & Frith, C. D. (1998). Differential activation of right superior parietal cortex and intraparietal sulcus by spatial and nonspatial attention. *NeuroImage, 8*, 176–187.

Coull, J. T., & Nobre, A. C. (1998). Where and when to pay attention: The neural systems for directing attention to spatial locations and to time intervals as revealed by both PET and fMRI. *Journal of Neuroscience, 18*, 7426–7435.

Cox, R. W. (1996). AFNI: Software for analysis and visualization of functional magnetic resonance neuroimages. *Computational Biomedical Research, 29*, 162–173.

Craver-Lemley, C., Arterberry, M. E., & Reeves, A. (1999). "Illusory" illusory conjunctions: The conjoining of features of visual and imagined stimuli. *Journal of Experimental Psychology: Human Perception and Performance, 25*, 1036–1049.

D'Esposito, M., Detre, J. A., Aguirre, G. K., Stallcup, M., Alsop, D. C., Tippet, L. J., & Farah, M. J. (1997). A functional MRI study of mental image generation. *Neuropsychologia, 35*, 725–730.

De Volder, A. G., Toyama, H., Kimura, Y., Kiyosawa, M., Nahano, H., Vanlierde, A., Wanet-Defalque, M.-C., Mishina, M., Oda, K., Ishiwata, K., & Senda, M. (2001). Auditory triggered mental imagery of shape involves visual association areas in early blind humans. *NeuroImage, 14*, 129–139.

Diwadkar, V. A., Carpenter, P. A., & Just, M. A. (2000). Collaborative activity between parietal and dorso-lateral prefrontal cortex in dynamic spatial working memory revealed by fMRI. *NeuroImage, 12*, 85–99.

Fallgatter, A. J., Mueller, T. J., & Strik, W. K. (1997). Neurophysiological correlates of mental imagery in different sensory modalities. *International Journal of Psychophysiology, 25*, 145–153.

Farah, M. J. (1995). Current issues in the neuropsychology of image generation. *Neuropsychologia, 33*, 1455–1471.

Farah, M. J. (2000). The neural bases of mental imagery. In M. S. Gazzaniga (Ed.), *The new cognitive neurosciences* (2nd ed., pp. 965–974). Cambridge, MA: MIT Press.

Farah, M. J., Weisberg, L. L., Monheit, M., & Peronnet, F. (1990). Brain activity underlying mental imagery: Event related potentials during mental image generation. *Journal of Cognitive Neuroscience, 1*, 302–316.

Farthing, C. W., Venturino, M., & Brown, S. W. (1983). Relationship between two different types of imagery vividness questionnaire items and three hypnotic susceptibility scale factors: A brief communication. *International Journal of Clinical and Experimental Hypnosis, 31*, 8–13.

Findlay, R., Ashton, R., & McFarland, K. (1994). Hemispheric differences in image generation and use in the haptic modality. *Brain and Cognition, 25*, 67–78.

Gilbert, A. N., Crouch, M., & Kemp, S. E. (1998). Olfactory and visual mental imagery. *Journal of Mental Imagery, 22*, 137–146.

Gissurarson, L. R. (1992). Reported auditory imagery and its relationship with visual imagery. *Journal of Mental Imagery, 16*, 117–122.

Goldenberg, G., Podreka, I., Steiner, M., & Willmes, K. (1987). Patterns of regional cerebral blood flow related to meaningfulness and imaginability of words—An emission computer tomography study. *Neuropsychologia, 25*, 473–486.

Goldman-Rakic, P. (2000). Localization of function all over again. *NeuroImage, 11*, 451–457.

Haxby, J. V., Hoewitz, B., Ungerleider, L. G., Maisog, J. M., Pietrini, P., & Grady, C. L. (1994). The functional organization of human extrastriate cortex: A PET-rCBF study of selective attention to faces and locations. *Journal of Neuroscience, 14*, 6336–6353.

Hishitani, S., & Murakami, S. (1992). What is vividness of imagery? Characteristics of vivid visual imagery. *Perceptual and Motor Skills, 75*, 1291–1307.

Höllinger, P., Beisteiner, R., Lang, W., Lindinger, G., & Berthoz, A. (1999). Mental representations of movements: Brain potentials associated with imagination of eye movements. *Clinical Neurophysiology, 110*, 799–805.

Isaac, A., Marks, D. F., & Russell, D. G. (1986). An instrument for assessing imagery of movement: The Vividness of Movement Imagery Questionnaire. *Journal of Mental Imagery, 10*, 23–30.

Ishai, A., Ungerleider, L. G., & Haxby, J. V. (2000). Distributed neural systems for the generation of visual images. *Neuron, 28*, 979–990.

Iwaki, S., Ueno, S., Imada, T., & Tonoike, M. (1999). Dynamic cortical activation in mental image processing revealed by biomagnetic measurement. *Neuroreport, 10*, 1793–1797.

Jeannerod, M. (1995). Mental imagery in the motor context. *Neuropsychologia, 33*, 1419–1432.

Jordan, K., Heinze, H.-J., Lutz, K., Kanowski, M., & Länche, L. (2001). Cortical activations during the mental rotation of different visual objects. *NeuroImage, 13*, 143–152.

Klein, I., Paradis, A.-L., Poline, J.-B., Kosslyn, S. M., & Le Bihan, D. (2000). Transient activity in the human calcarine cortex during visual mental imagery: An event-related fMRI study. *Journal of Cognitive Neuroscience, 12*, 15–23.

Kosslyn, S. M. (1994). *Image and brain: The resolution of the imagery debate*. Cambridge, MA: MIT Press.

Kosslyn, S. M., Alpert, N. M., Thompson, W. L., Maljkovic, V., Weise, S. B., Chabris, C. F., Hamilton, S. E., Rauch, S. L., & Buonanno, F. S. (1993). Visual mental imagery activates topographically organized visual areas: PET investigations. *Journal of Cognitive Neuroscience, 5*, 263–287.

Kosslyn, S. M., & Rabin, C. (1999). The representation of left–right orientation: A dissociation between imagery and perceptual recognition. *Visual Cognition, 6*, 497–508.

Kosslyn, S. M., & Thompson, W. L. (2000). Shared mechanisms in visual imagery and visual perception: Insights from cognitive neuroscience. In M. S. Gazzaniga (Ed.), *The new cognitive neurosciences* (2nd ed., pp. 975–985). Cambridge, MA: MIT Press.

Kosslyn, S. M., Thompson, W. L., Kim, I. J., & Alpert, N. M. (1995). Topographical representations of mental images in primary visual cortex. *Nature, 378*, 496–498.

Lehman, D., Kochi, K., Koenig, T., Koykkou, M., Michel, C. M., & Strik, W. K. (1994). Microstates of the brain electric field and momentary mind states. In M. Eiselt, U. Zwiener, & H. Witte

(Eds.), *Quantitative and topological EEG and MEG analysis*. Jena, Germany: Universitätsverlag Mayer.

Levine, D. N., Warach, J., & Farah, M. J. (1985). Two visual systems in mental imagery: Dissociation of "what" and "where" in imagery disorders due to bilateral posterior cerebral lesions. *Neurology, 35*, 1010–1018.

Marks, D. F. (1989). Bibliography of research utilizing the Vividness of Visual Imagery Questionnaire. *Perceptual and Motor Skills, 69*, 707–718.

Marks, D. F., & Isaac, A. R. (1995). Topographical distribution of EEG activity accompanying visual and motor imagery in vivid and non-vivid imagers. *British Journal of Psychology, 86*, 271–282.

Mellet, E., Petit, L., Mazoyer, B. M., Denis, M., & Tzourio-Mazoyer, N. (1998a). Reopening the mental imagery debate: Lessons from functional anatomy. *NeuroImage, 8*, 2129–2139.

Mellet, E., Tzourio-Mazoyer, N., Bricogne, S., Mazoyer, B. M., Kosslyn, S. M., & Denis, M. (2000). Functional anatomy of high-resolution visual mental imagery. *Journal of Cognitive Neuroscience, 12*, 98–109.

Mellet, E., Tzourio-Mazoyer, N., Crivello, F., Joliot, M., Denis, M., & Mazoyer, B. M. (1996). Functional anatomy of spatial mental imagery generated from verbal instruction. *Journal of Neuroscience, 16*, 6504–6512.

Mellet, E., Tzourio-Mazoyer, N., Denis, M., & Mazoyer, B. M. (1998b). Cortical anatomy of mental imagery of concrete nouns based on their dictionary definition. *Neuroreport, 9*, 803–808.

Miller, E. K. (2000). The prefrontal cortex: No simple matter. *NeuroImage, 11*, 447–450.

Miyashita, Y. (1995). How the brain creates imagery: Projections to the primary visual cortex. *Science, 23*, 1719–1720.

Olivetti Belardinelli, M., Di Matteo, R., Del Gratta, C., De Nicola, A., Ferretti, A., & Romani, G. L. (2004). Commonalities between visual imagery and imagery in other modalities: An investigation by means of fMRI. In E. Carsetti (Ed.), *Seeing, thinking and knowing* (pp. 203–218). Dordrecht, The Netherlands: Kluwer Academic Publishers.

Owen, A. M., Evans, A. C., & Petrides, M. (1996). Evidence for a two-stage model of spatial working memory processing within the lateral frontal cortex: A positron emission tomography study. *Cerebral Cortex, 6*, 61–38.

Petsche, H., Lacroix, D., Lindner, K., Rappelsberger, P., & Schmidt, H. E. (1992). Thinking with images or thinking with language: A pilot EEG probability mapping study. *International Journal of Psychophysiology, 12*, 31–39.

Porro, C. A., Francescato, M. P., Cettolo, V., Diamond, M. E., Baraldi, P., Zuiani, C., Bazzocchi, M., & Di Prampero, P. E. (1996). Primary motor and sensory cortex activation during motor performance and motor imagery: A functional magnetic resonance study. *Journal of Neuroscience, 16*, 7688–7698.

Rao, S. M., Bandettini, P. A., Hammeke, T. A., Yetkin, F. Z., Jesmanowicz, A., Lisk, L. M., Morris, G. L., Mueller, W. M., Estkowski, L. D., Wong, E. C., Haughton, V. M., & Hyde, J. S. (1993). Functional magnetic resonance imaging of complex human movements. *Neurology, 43*, 2311–2318.

Roth, M., Decety, J., Raybaudi, M., Massarelli, R., Delon-Martin, C., Segebarth, C., Morand, S., Gemignani, A., Décorps, M., & Jeannerod, M. (1996). Possible involvement of primary motor cortex in mentally simulated movements: A functional magnetic resonance imaging study. *Neuroreport, 7*, 1280–1284.

Rugg, M. D. (1997). Introduction. In M. D. Rugg (Ed.), *Cognitive neuroscience* (2nd ed., pp. 1–9). Hove, UK: Psychology Press.

Rushworth, M. F. S., & Owen, A. M. (1998). The functional organization of the lateral frontal cortex: Conjecture or conjuncture in the electrophysiology literature? *Trends in Cognitive Science, 2*, 46–53.

Savic, I. (2001). Processing of odorous signals in humans. *Brain Research Bulletin, 54*, 307–312.

Sheehan, P. W. (1967). A shortened form of Betts' questionnaire upon mental imagery. *Journal of Clinical Psychology, 23*, 386–389.

Spector, A. C. (2000). Linking gustatory neurobiology to behavior in vertebrates. *Neuroscience and Biobehavioral Reviews, 24*, 391–416.

Stephan, K. M., Fink, G. R., Passingham, R. E., Silbersweig, D., Ceballos-Baumann, A. O., Frith, C. D., & Frackowiak, R. S. J. (1995). Functional anatomy of the mental representations of upper extremity movements in healthy subjects. *Journal of Neurophysiology, 73*, 373–386.

Stewart, L., Meyer, B.-U., Frith, U., & Rothwell, J. (2001). Left posterior BA37 is involved in object recognition: A TMS study. *Neuropsychologia, 39*, 1–6.

Thomas, N. J. T. (1999). Are theories of imagery theories of imagination? An active perception approach to conscious mental content. *Cognitive Science, 23*, 207–245.

Thompson, W. L., Kosslyn, S. M., Sukel, K. E., & Alpert, N. M. (2001). Mental imagery of high- and low-resolution gratings activates area 17. *NeuroImage, 14*, 454–464.

Thompson-Schill, S. L., Aguirre, G. K., D'Esposito, M., & Farah, M. J. (1999). A neural basis for category and modality specificity of semantic knowledge. *Neuropsychologia, 37*, 671–676.

White, K. D., Ashton, R., & Brown, R. M. D. (1977). The measurement of imagery vividness: Normative data and their relationship to sex, age, and modality differences. *British Journal of Psychology, 68*, 203–211.

Wilson, F. A. W., Ó Scalaidhe, S. P., & Goldman-Rakic, P. S. (1993). Dissociations of object and spatial processing domains in primate prefrontal cortex. *Science, 260*, 1955–1958.

Wise, R. J. S., Howard, D., Mummery, C. J., Fletcher, P., Leff, A., Büchel, C., & Scott, S. K. (2000). Noun imageability and the temporal lobes. *Neuropsychologia, 38*, 958–994.

Wolpin, M., & Weinstein, C. (1983). Visual imagery and olfactory stimulation. *Journal of Mental Imagery, 7*, 63–74.

Yamamoto, S., & Mukai, H. (1998). Event-related potentials during mental imagery. *Neuroreport, 9*, 3359–3362.

Zald, D. H., & Pardo, J. V. (2000). Functional neuroimaging of the olfactory system in humans. *International Journal of Psychophysiology, 36*, 165–181.

Zatorre, R. J., & Halpern, A. R. (1993). Effect of unilateral temporal-lobe excision on perception and imagery of songs. *Neuropsychologia, 31*, 221–232.

Zatorre, R. J., Halpern, A. R., Perry, D. W., Meyer, E., & Evans, A. C. (1996). Hearing in the mind's ear: A PET investigation of musical imagery and perception. *Journal of Cognitive Neuroscience, 8*, 29–46.

EUROPEAN JOURNAL OF COGNITIVE PSYCHOLOGY, 2004, *16* (5), 753–766

Visuospatial representations used by chess experts: A preliminary study

Pertti Saariluoma

Computer and Information Sciences, University of Jyväskylä, Finland

Hasse Karlsson

Department of Psychiatry, University of Helsinki, and PET Centre, University Central Hospital of Turku, Finland

Heikki Lyytinen

Department of Psychology, University of Jyväskylä, Finland

Mika Teräs and Fabian Geisler

PET Centre, University Central Hospital of Turku, Finland

Blindfold chess is played without the players seeing either the pieces or the board. It is a skill-related activity, and only very skilled players can construct the mental images required. This is why blindfold chess provides a good task with which to investigate the spatial memory and skilled mental images of expert players. In a PET investigation, we compared memory performance and problem solving in very experienced chess players with their performance in an attention task, in which the subjects classified the names of chess pieces. The memory task predominantly activated the temporal areas, whereas problem solving activated several frontal areas. The relevance of these findings to concepts such as general imagery, skilled imagery, apperception, and long-term working memory are discussed.

Understanding the cognitive structure associated with tasks is one prerequisite for understanding the neural frameworks of mental processes. Chess is a particularly interesting domain from this perspective. It is also important to vary the way basic concepts such as mental imagery are operationalised to avoid the

Correspondence should be addressed to Pertti Saariluoma, Computer and Information Sciences, University of Jyväskylä, Box 35, Jyväskylä, Finland. Email: psa@it.jyu.fi

This work was funded by the University of Helsinki for the first author, and by the Turku PET Centre. We would like to thank Steven Crawford for correcting the English. We also thank Michel Denis and two anonymous reviewers for very detailed and constructive comments.

© 2004 Psychology Press Ltd
http://www.tandf.co.uk/journals/pp/09541446.html   DOI:10.1080/09541440340000501

metascientific "Ebbinghaus effect", i.e., using materials that are too abstract and produce too narrow stimuli, and thus unintentionally overlooking some essential aspects of basic theoretical concepts (see Saariluoma, 1997).

For many decades, chess has been used as the "fruit fly" of expertise research. For many reasons, it is a suitable platform for this kind of basic research. It is a genuine problem-solving domain, and people have often used their free time for years to learn to play it. It is also easy to measure the level of skill in chess, which enables us to obtain a clear idea about the level of performance of the subjects (Charness, 1976, 1992; de Groot, 1965, 1966; de Groot & Gobet, 1996; Newell & Simon, 1972; Saariluoma, 1995). Chess therefore seems to be a good domain for investigating the use of mental images.

Chess imagery is not of interest for what it tells us about the game itself, but because it provides us with information about a specific type of mental imagery. These images can be called "skilled images", because the ability to construct such images develops with increasing expertise. Naturally, this kind of imagery is vital in many practical environments, because there is a multitude of professions in which skilled images are essential. These images typically have a very complex structure, and cannot be represented by a single scene. In the domain of chess, such images may entail hundreds of moves, and over 10,000 piece locations (Saariluoma, 1991, 1995). Nevertheless, to date we have relatively little information about the specific properties of such images.

Two sets of consistent experimental evidence support the lay intuition that chess players rely on mental images when playing (Abrahams, 1951; Krogius, 1976). Firstly, research on chess players' recall of visually presented chess positions supports the relevance of imagery processes in storing chess-specific information (de Groot, 1965, 1966; Djakov, Petrovsky, & Rudik, 1926). The main finding, which was obtained by Lemmens and Jongman (unpublished; see Vicente & de Groot, 1990), has undoubtedly been the well-known interaction between a player's skill level and the types of positions (de Groot & Gobet, 1996; Gobet, 1998; Gobet & Simon, 1996; Saariluoma, 1995, 2001).

The interaction between skill and position type has subsequently been replicated several times (e.g., Chase & Simon, 1973a, 1973b; Frey & Adesman, 1976; Saariluoma, 1985, 1994, 1998; Vicente, 1988). As is well known, this phenomenon has been found to be important in the theory of human long-term working memory and cognitive skills (Ericsson & Kintsch, 1995; Saariluoma, 1995; Vicente, 1988). Moreover, recent experiments have shown the importance of the so-called absolute location of chess chunks, i.e., the impaired recall of chess chunks when transformed into incorrect locations on a chessboard. These empirical findings highlight the importance of the spatial character of chunking in chess (Gobet & Simon, 1996; Saariluoma, 1994).

Secondly, investigations of chess memory also suggest that visual imagery is a very active processing resource in chess players' thinking (for reviews, see e.g., Gobet & Simon, 1996; de Groot & Gobet, 1996; Lemmens & Jongman, unpublished, see Vicente & de Groot, 1990; Saariluoma, 1995, 2001; Vicente & de Groot, 1990). Empirical investigations of chess players' perceptual processes have demonstrated that mental transformation plays an important role in chess players' thinking (Bachmann & Oit, 1992; Chase & Simon, 1973a, 1973b; Church & Church, 1977; Milojkovic, 1982; Saariluoma, 1985). Working memory studies have systematically implied the active use of the visuospatial memory during the processing of chess-specific information (Baddeley, 1983, 1986; Baddeley & Hitch, 1974; Robbins et al., 1995; Saariluoma, 1989, 1991, 1992c).

Blindfold chess experiments have also provided information about the functions of imagery in chess. In blindfold chess, players do not see the board or the pieces, and the opponent's moves are given by using the names of the pieces and their board coordinates (e.g., "bishop from c4 to f7"). Consequently, blindfold players must rely entirely on their visual memory and mental imagery when playing. They sometimes play several games simultaneously (Cleveland, 1907; Holding, 1985; Wason's first comment in Binet, 1893/1966).

Blindfold chess is a highly skill-related ability. The more skilled a player is, the better he or she normally plays blindfold chess (Saariluoma, 1991; Saariluoma & Kalakoski, 1997, 1998). The memory load involved can be substantial. In our experiments, subjects successfully followed the verbal reading of 10 different games simultaneously, involving up to 70 responses (Saariluoma, 1991). All this suggests that blindfold chess is a good domain in which to investigate the psychological properties of mental images.

An interesting problem is the neural representation of chess players' mental images. This information is important for several reasons. It can tell us about the resources required for building skilled and complex images, that is, images that only experts can generate, and that cannot be represented as a single scene (Saariluoma, 1989, 1991, 1995, 2001; Saariluoma & Kalakoski, 1997, 1998). It can also enable us to consider the neural representations of long-term working memory, because it is evident that chess-specific information in memory tasks must be passed into this area of storage.

Finally, we can also discuss the neural resources required in apperception (e.g., Saariluoma, 1990, 1992b, 1995, 2001). When people construct mental representations, contents of these representations almost always entail elements that cannot be reduced to the physically perceivable environment. As perception and attention are stimulus-bound processes (i.e., we cannot perceive anything that has no direct relationship to the retinal image and thus to the physically present environment), it is necessary to assume nonstimulus bound mental operations. Closing one's eyes eliminates perceptual, but not mental representations. Apperception, as the process of constructing mental representations, is of course a phenomenon of this nature (Kant, 1787; Leibniz, 1704/1979; Stout, 1896; Wundt, 1880). Especially interesting here is the relationship of mental images to apperception, because imagery processes are not bound to the physical presence of stimuli.

At the moment, we have relatively little information about the brain mechanisms underlying chess players' information processing (Charness, 1988; Cranberg & Albert, 1988). An especially interesting study is that of Nichelli, Grafman, Pietrini, Alway, Carton, and Miletich (1994). In this PET research, the main aim was to investigate the brain activity associated with chess playing to get an idea of the neural representations involved in such a complex cognitive skill. Four conditions were used, where chess diagrams were visually presented to the subjects on a computer screen. In the first condition, the participants had to say whether a piece of a given colour was on the board (during this task, Brodmann's Areas 7 and 19 were active); in the second, they had to say which piece was nearest to a given mark (Areas 6 and 7 were active in this case); in the third, the subjects answered a question about whether one piece could take another or not (activations were found in the hippocampus and the temporal lobe); finally, the subjects had to decide whether a one-move mate was possible or not (Areas 7, 18, and 19 were activated). The main finding of this experiment was that complex problem solving called for the concerted activation of a network of several interrelated, but functionally distinct, cerebral areas.

In the research referred to, we concentrated on two main experimental presuppositions. These were the relatively low-level chess-specific task demands and the visual presentation of the tasks. Only the last two tasks required chess-playing skill, although they were relatively easy for any experienced chess player. Certainly, the tasks used provided us with solid data about chess skill, but it should be possible to construct substantially more difficult tasks. One possibility is to use blindfold chess.

We decided to use three different types of chess-specific tasks. In all of them, the basic information was communicated auditorily. This was done to distinguish between visual images and chess-specific visual perception. It is known that there is substantial, but not complete, overlap between visual images and percepts in the brain (Farah, 1985; Finke, 1985; Kosslyn, 1980, 1994; Saariluoma, 1992a). Here, we thought it would be reasonable to eliminate the visual input as far as possible and concentrate on "pure" mental imagery. Auditory presentation provides a way of doing this, and the subjects really have to construct spatial images without relying on the visual input of a chessboard as an external memory.

The three experimental conditions consisted of tasks that made increasing demands for processing resources. In the first task, subjects had to use their auditory attention to identify target piece names; in the second, they had to remember games in which the moves were described verbally to them; and in the third, they had to play blindfold chess, in which the moves were also described verbally to them. These tasks were termed attention, memory, and problem solving, respectively. The first task was used as a baseline, and we looked for the brain areas in which brain activity was greater during the other two tasks.

Specifically, we assumed that the memory – attention comparison would provide us with information about mental imagery and the storage of complex spatial information, whereas the problem solving – attention comparison would provide information about neural resources involved in both storing information and moving pieces over the imagined board. Finally, the problem solving – memory comparison could be expected to provide information about supervisory control systems or central executive-type planning control mechanisms, which must play an important role in the apperceptive construction of representations.

METHOD

Subjects

Six experienced chess players took part in the experiment. Their mean SELO grading was 2084 points, and they had an average of 37 years of experience of competitive chess. They were all right-handed men. The SELO grading is a measure of chess players' strength. It is calculated on the basis of their competitive success as a measure of skill, and is thus an objective measure. The mean SELO rating is 1750 and the standard deviation 200 points. This means that, on average, the subjects had a skill level score around 2 standard deviations above the mean for competitive chess players in Finland. The SELO measure is equivalent to the international ELO rating system (Elo, 1978). The mean age of the subjects was over 45. They were all under 60. Subject 6 was dropped, because, although he was a chess master, he could not play blindfold chess. He told us that he had never experienced any mental images of any kind in his life. We report the analysis of his results in another context.

Design and procedure

This research was approved by the Ethics Committee of the University of Turku. Subjects were presented with three chess-specific blindfold tasks.

In the attention task, they were provided with the names of chess pieces (e.g., black queen, white pawn, etc.) in random order from a tape recorder at a speed of one piece name every 4 s. The task of the subjects was to raise the forefinger of their right hand every time they heard a minor piece (i.e., bishop or knight) in the sequence.

In the memory task, the subjects had to follow games read from a tape (half moves, i.e., a move by white or a move by black, e.g., "knight g1–f3"). The speed was also one move every 4 s. The task of the participants was to memorise the read-out games and to repeat them to the experimenter if asked later. This was not actually done for technical reasons, but the subjects did not know that it wouldn't be. All the subjects said that they had a normal memory representation of the positions.

In the problem-solving task, the subjects were asked to play blindfolded against a chess computer program (Fritz). In this task, the moves of Fritz were described to them verbally by the experimenter (e.g., "e2–e4"). The subjects had the white pieces. If they lost the game before the session was over, they were asked to begin a new one. Here the speed of presentation was free and depended on the subjects. All the subjects must have been able to remember the positions, because otherwise they would have been unable to make logical moves. The order in which the three conditions were presented was balanced across the six subjects.

All the subjects were positioned in a PET scanner. Three different measurements were made per condition, and so including the transmission scan, the total number of measurements recorded was 10. In each condition, the first measurement was started after 4 min and the next two at 8 min intervals. After the third measurement for one condition, the next experimental condition began after an interval of 1–2 min. The total duration of the experimental sessions was around one-and-a-half hours.

Before the experiment, the subjects were instructed to avoid thinking of moves during the attention conditions. In the poblem-solving conditions, they were told when the measurements began. This was related to the nature of blindfold chess. The blindfold players made their moves verbally, and we wanted to avoid forcing the activation of speech centres and also to minimise the possibility of head movements. Some activation naturally might remain, but there were no unnecessary head movements. Playing chess with a computer is a complex problem-solving task with a creative content.

PET imaging technique

O-15-labelled water was produced by a Cyclone 3 low-energy deuteron accelerator (Ion Beam Application, Inc., Louvain-la-Neuve, Belgium). Cyclone 3 is a compact cyclotron for hospital use, and it accelerates positively charged deuteron ions up to 3.8 MeV to generate O-15-labelled compounds for PET applications. The O-15 water was produced by a dialysis technique in a continuously working water module (Clark, Crouzel, Meyer, & Strijckmans, 1987). O-15 has a half-life of 123 s. Sterility and pyrogen tests were performed to confirm the purity of the product.

We obtained rCBF scans for each individual subject by using a GE Advance PET Scanner (General Motors Medical Systems, Milwaukee, WI, USA). This apparatus has been described in detail in Lewellen, Kohlmyer, Miyaoka, Kaplan, Stearns, and Schubert (1996). It has 18 detector rings with 672 crystals/ring (6 × 6 blocks), and provides 35 transverse sections through the brain spaced 4.25 mm apart (centre to centre/axial sampling interval) covering 152 mm axially (axial field of view) and with an aperture of 550 mm. The transmission scan performed with a Ge-68/Ga-68 source was used for measured attenuation correction. The head of the subject was positioned correctly using a laser-positioning system according to the cantho-meatal reference line. A filtered back-projection algo-rithm was employed to reconstruct the image on a 128 × 128 matrix.

The regional cerebral blood flow (rCBF) during each task was measured by recording the distribution of radioactivity in the brain following an IV injection of 250 MBq of O-15-labelled water through a forearm cannula. According to the current guidelines of the Turku PET Centre, nine tasks were attempted per subject. The minimum interval between the O-15 water injections was 8 min. For each of the nine scans, the task began 4 min before the intravenous bolus (10 ml in 10–15 s) of 250 MBq O-15 water was administered. After the injection of the O-15 water, data were acquired in 3D mode for 90 s, starting when the tracer entered the brain, for which the criterion was a true coincidence rate over the threshold of 15,000 counts/s. The data were framed into a single 90 s static frame (Holm, Law, & Paulson, 1996; Laine, Rinne, Krause, Teräs, & Sipilä, 1999).

Analysis of the data

The data were first transformed into the ANALYZE format using a converter program especially developed for this purpose at the Turku PET Centre. The actual quantitative analysis of the 90s images was carried out using the Statis-tical Parametric Mapping software (SPM 99, The Wellcome Department of Cognitive Neurology, London, UK; Friston, Ashburner, Frith, Poline, Heather, & Frackowiak, 1995a; Friston, Holmes, Worsley, Poline, Frith, & Frackowiak, 1995b). Each reconstructed O-15-water scan was realigned according to the bicommissural line into a stereotactic space corresponding to the atlas of Talairach and Tournoux (1988) using a PET template, and normalised according to Friston et al. (1995a). A Gaussian filter with a half-maximum full width (15 mm) was applied to smooth each image to compensate for intersubject differ-ences and to suppress high frequency noise in the images. Differences in global activity within and between subjects were removed by the analysis of covariance (ANCOVA) on a voxel by voxel basis, with global counts as covariates of regional activity across subjects for each task. This was because inter- and intrasubject differences in global activity may obscure regional alterations in activity following cognitive stimulation. For each pixel in stereotactic space, the ANCOVA generated a condition-specific, adjusted mean rCBF value (normal-ised to 50 ml/100 ml per min), and an associated adjusted error variance. The ANCOVA made it possible to compare the means across the different conditions using t statistics. The resulting map of t values constituted a statistical para-metric map (Friston et al., 1995a).

RESULTS AND DISCUSSION

The statistically significant outcomes of an SPM analysis (ANCOVA, $p < .001$, uncorrected, voxel size = 2.0 × 2.0 × 2.0 mm) are shown in Figure 1, where memory and problem solving are compared to attention, and problem solving is

(a)

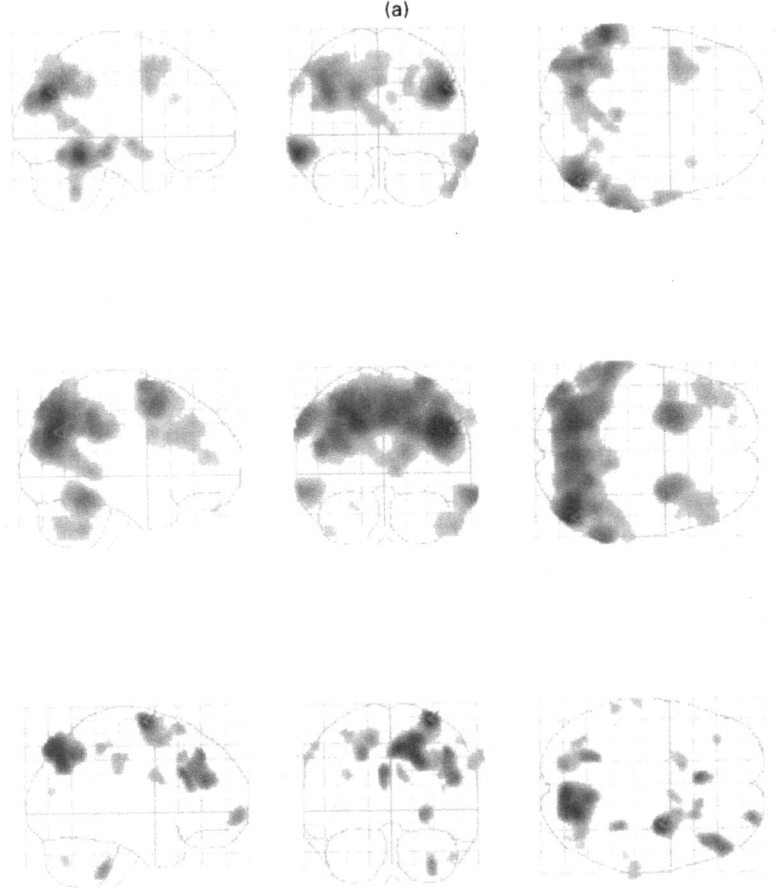

Figure 1. Brain regions associated with blindfold chess. **(a)** Memory – Attention; **(b)** Problem solving – Attention; **(c)** Problem solving – Memory.

compared to memory. The data collected in the attention task were used as a baseline.

A more detailed presentation of the findings can be seen in Table 1. It enables us to make systematic comparisons with the findings of other relevant experimental investigations.

Before discussing the interpretation and making comparisons with the data reported by others, it is necessary to point out some specific characteristics of images in chess. The most important characteristic is naturally that blindfold chess is not something that can be done by everyone. One really has to have

TABLE 1

Stereotactic coordinates, anatomical localisations of the activations, Brodmann's Areas (BA), and local maxima Z scores, in the three comparisons (ANCOVA uncorrected; t values corrected for entire volume)

Comparison	MNI coordinates (x, y, z)			Talairach coordinates (x, y, z)			Anatomical localisation	BA	k	t values	Z scores
Memory – Attention											
1	52,	−72,	36	51.5,	−68.1,	36.6	G. angularis	39	1808	7.85	5.86
2	−62,	−48,	14	−61.4,	−47.1,	−9.4	G. tempor. inf.	37	1305	7.41	5.65
3	−40,	−70,	36	−39.6,	−66.2,	36.5	G. angularis	39/19	4941	6.08	4.95
4	70,	−44,	−18	69.3,	−43.4,	−13.0	G. tempor. inf.	37	1026	5.72	4.73
5	68,	−8,	−6	67.3,	−8.0,	−4.6	G. tempor. medius	21	269	4.81	4.16
6	−36,	6,	54	−35.6,	8.3,	49.3	G. front. medius	6	1116	4.77	4.13
7	0,	−40,	42	0.0,	−36.8,	40.5	G. cinguli	31	122	4.62	4.03
8	40,	16,	54	39.6,	18.0,	48.8	G. front. medius	8	52	3.96	3.55
Problem solving – Attention											
1	52,	−72,	34	51.5,	−68.2,	34.7	G. angularis	39	19411	10.12	6.78
2	70,	−48,	−18	69.3,	−47.3,	−12.8	G. tempor. inf.	37	1607	9.68	6.62
3	−26,	6,	58	−25.7,	8.5,	53.0	G. front. medius	6	2215	7.72	5.80
4	32,	0,	68	32.7,	3.1,	62.5	G. front. sup.	6	2678	7.02	5.46
5	−62,	−50,	−14	−61.4,	−49.0,	−9.3	G. tempor. inf.	37	761	6.59	5.23
6	−42,	34,	32	−41.6,	34.4,	27.8	G. front. medius	9	573	5.05	4.31
7	−38,	48,	14	−37.6,	47.1,	10.5	G. front. medius	10	188	4.14	3.70
8	−42,	−50,	−48	−41.6,	−50.5,	−37.8	Cerebellum		44	3.79	3.43
9	−26,	52,	−26	−25.7,	49.3,	−24.3	G. front. sup.	11	10	3.54	3.24
Problem solving – Memory											
1	30,	−8,	70	29.7,	−4.5,	59.1	G. front. sup.	6	724	5.34	4.50
2	6,	−80,	46	5.9,	−75.4,	46.1	Precuneus	7	1965	5.16	4.39
3	44,	36,	44	43.6,	36.7,	35.2	G. front. medius	9	608	4.76	4.12
4	−6,	24,	28	−5.9,	24.5,	24.6	G. cinguli	24	163	4.76	4.12
5	−22,	−62,	44	−21.8,	−58.0,	43.4	Precuneus	7	677	4.50	3.95
6	26,	64,	−2	25.7,	61.9,	−4.8	G. front. sup.	10	142	4.32	3.82
7	32,	−40,	−44	31.7,	−40.8,	−38.5	Cerebellum		118	4.25	3.77
8	16,	22,	42	15.8,	23.2,	37.5	G. front. medius	32	66	3.93	3.53
9	70,	−28,	42	69.3,	−25.2,	40.0	G. postcentralis	2	116	3.88	3.50

been trained in chess. This is different from many neuroimaging studies of mental images.

Our subjects displayed strong automation and large patterns of chess specific knowledge. This is quite normal in skills research, but it operationalises the notion of mental imagery very differently from tasks that can be done by ordinary people without training. Chess also assumes very complex information processing compared to small matrices or other relatively abstract and elementary stimuli (see e.g., Newell & Simon, 1972, or Saariluoma, 1995, about the properties of chess).

In the attention task, people need only encode word meanings. The spatial demands are minimal, because no spatial information about the locations of the pieces is given. The names of the pieces are also highly automated in the minds of people with an experience level of around 35 years of practice. The memory task is much more spatial, because one has to store the locations of the pieces and their movements. It also presupposes long-term working memory storage with spatial encoding (Ericsson & Kintsch, 1995; Saariluoma & Kalakoski, 1997, 1998). Finally, chess players' problem solving requires mental transformation of the pieces (Chase & Simon, 1973a, 1973b; de Groot, 1965; de Groot & Gobet, 1996; Saariluoma, 1995). In addition, it implies conceptual abstraction and the selection of a few relevant possibilities among millions of alternatives, which is essentially apperceiving (Saariluoma, 1990, 1995, 2001).

An important question in recent imagery research has been the sharing of neural resources between percepts and images (Cocude, Mellet, & Denis, 1999; Farah, 1985; Kosslyn, 1994; Mellet, Tzourio-Mazoyer, Bricogne, Mazoyer, Kosslyn, & Denis, 2000; Moscovitch, Behrmann, & Winocur, 1994; Saariluoma, 1992a). Our investigation does not show any activity in the primary visual areas. The obvious explanation is the fact that the earlier studies used visual presentation whereas in this study we used auditory presentation of the information. Interestingly, we know that auditorily presented information in chess is transferred into a visuospatial format, and that the visuospatial working memory has systematically been shown to be involved in the processing of chess materials (Robbins et al., 1995; Saariluoma, 1989, 1991, 1992c, 1995; Saariluoma & Kalakoski, 1997, 1998). Hence, primary perceptual areas seem to play a minor role in processing chess-specific images. In addition, the outcome suggests that the visuospatial memory does not essentially rely on the primary visual cortex.

The crucial difference between the attention and memory tasks is in the storage demands they make. The attention task does not presuppose any spatial information storage, whereas the memory task does. If we subtract attention from memory, we should get a good idea of the resources required to store such spatial, automatised, and expertise-demanding materials as chess positions.

The gyrus angularis (area 39) is active on both sides in the memory task. There is a set of similar findings from the earlier neuroimaging experiments on imagery, but activation of this area is often absent (Cabeza & Nyberg, 2000). Mellet et al. (2000), for example, did not find such activation. This area is often associated with hearing other people's speech and auditory associations (Cabeza & Nyberg, 2000; Talairach & Tournoux, 1988). Undoubtedly, the method we used to present information could be one explanation for this activation.

We found also activation in the inferior and medial temporal cortex, in Areas 37 and 21. The latter is located on the right side, and the former on both sides. Area 37 has been found to be active, for instance, when listening to texts

(Cabeza & Nyberg, 2000; see also Mellet et al., 2000). Cabeza and Nyberg have reported in their review that Area 21 is very commonly laterally active in imagery tasks. Area 31 is activated in the middle and Area 8 is activated on the right, whereas Area 6 is activated on the left. The first area is only uncommonly found in imagery studies, whereas the latter is rather commonly detected. Finally, we recorded activation of the gyrus frontalis medius, as some other authors have (cf. Cabeza & Nyberg, 2000).

Comparing our study with that of Mellet et al. (2000), we find that there is overall similarity between our findings (with temporal, parietal, and frontal activations), but there are also differences. The comparison suggests that there is a substantial neural difference between elementary forms of images and complex skilled images (for skilled images, see Saariluoma, 1991; Saariluoma & Kalakoski, 1997, 1998). Automatisation is one possible explanation. On the grounds of a general understanding of chess, the activated areas are likely to be relevant when neural correlates for long-term working memory are considered.

The next comparison was between attention and problem solving. The difference between task demands is different from the memory – attention difference, when additional processing is required in the main task. Problem solving in blindfold conditions involves storing information in the long-term working memory, but it also involves thinking-related activities such as planning and conceptual information processing (de Groot, 1965; de Groot & Gobet, 1996; Saariluoma, 1995). This is why we should expect increased activity in the frontal areas.

The areas activated are mostly the same as in the previous task, i.e., Areas 39, 37, and 9. This is understandable, because blindfold playing presupposes the same basic memory resources as following a game played by another person. These areas are relevant in long-term working memory activities (Ericsson & Kintsch, 1995). In addition, the areas mentioned are also partly shared with those detected in the memory – attention comparison, but clearly increased activity was also found in Area 6. This area is close to the frontal eye fields, which were found to be important in mental rotation by Just, Carpenter, Maguire, Diwadkar, and McMains (2001). These findings suggest that Area 6 is involved in the mental transformations necessary for searching in chess.

The main difference was increased frontal activity, which was naturally to be expected, but the activation of Areas 10 and 11 on the left was the main finding. The activation of Areas 10 and 11 was to be expected, since it has long been known that prefrontal cortical areas are important in planning and semantic memory processes (Cabeza & Nyberg, 2000). Both types of processes are relevant in chess players' apperceptive processes such as thinking and conceptualising (Saariluoma, 1995). Interestingly, imagery findings are rare, and Just et al. (2001), for example, did not record any activity in this area in a mental rotation task. In addition, we recorded increased activity in the cerebellum, which seems to have a role in the spatial working memory (Fiez, 2001).

Finally, we subtracted memory from problem solving to investigate areas that are relevant in controlling searching in problem spaces. The areas that are essential for keeping chess positions in mind should not be activated. This means that we should record an activity in the frontal areas, but temporal areas such as 36 and 37 should be less active. As one could expect, the activity differences in frontal areas were substantial. Areas 9, 10, and 24, which are all relevant in such frontal activities as planning and action control (Cabeza & Nyberg, 2000; Shallice, 2002), were activated. We can conclude that these areas are relevant in investigating neural correlates for apperceptive processes (Saariluoma, 1990, 1995, 2001).

To summarise, when we compare our results with the earlier findings concerning mental images, there are some similarities, and also some substantial differences. This suggests that chess experts' chess-specific images are not necessarily represented in the same way as ordinary mental images. From earlier cognitive work, we know that chess players' visuospatial representations are characterised by large prelearned visuospatial chunks and automated processing habits. This is presumably why these skilled images are in many respects different from ordinary images. The findings also provide us with valuable information about possible neural correlates of two important new concepts: long-term working memory and apperceptive processes (Ericsson & Kintsch, 1995; Saariluoma, 1990, 1995, 2001).

PrEview proof published online May 2004

REFERENCES

Abrahams, G. (1951). *The chess mind*. Harmondsworth, UK: Penguin Books.

Bachmann, T., & Oit, M. (1992). Stroop-like interference in chess players' imagery: An unexplored possibility to be revealed by the adapted moving-spot task. *Psychological Research, 54*, 27–31.

Baddeley, A. D. (1983). Working memory. *Philosophical Transactions of the Royal Society of London, Series B, 302*, 311–324.

Baddeley, A. D. (1986). *Working memory*. Cambridge, UK: Cambridge University Press.

Baddeley, A. D., & Hitch, G. (1974). Working memory. In G. H. Bower (Ed.), *The psychology of learning and motivation* (Vol. 8, pp. 47–89). New York: Academic Press.

Binet, A. (1966). Mnemonic virtuosity: A study of chess players. *Genetic Psychology Monographs, 74*, 127–164. (Original work published 1893.)

Cabeza, R., & Nyberg, L. (2000). Imaging and cognition: II. An empirical review of 275 PET and fMRI studies. *Journal of Cognitive Neuroscience, 12*, 1–47.

Charness, N. (1976). Memory for chess positions: Resistance to interference. *Journal of Experimental Psychology: Human Learning and Memory, 2*, 641–653.

Charness, N. (1988). Expertise in chess, music, and physics: A cognitive perspective. In L. Obler & D. Fein (Eds.), *The exceptional brain: Neuropsychology of talent and special abilities* (pp. 399–426). New York: Guilford.

Charness, N. (1992). The impact of chess research on cognitive science. *Psychological Research, 54*, 4–9.

Chase, W. G., & Simon, H. A. (1973a). Perception in chess. *Cognitive Psychology, 4*, 55–81.

Chase, W. G., & Simon, H. A. (1973b). The mind's eye in chess. In W. G. Chase (Ed.), *Visual information processing* (pp. 215–281). New York: Academic Press.

Church, R. M., & Church, K. W. (1977). Plans, goals, and search strategies for the selection of a move in chess. In P. W. Frey (Ed.), *Chess skill in man and machine.* New York: Springer.

Clark, J. C., Crouzel, C., Meyer, G. J., & Strijckmans, K. (1987). Current methodology for oxygen-15 production for clinical use. *Applied Radiation and Isotopes, 38,* 597–600.

Cleveland, A. A. (1907). The psychology of chess. *American Journal of Psychology, 18,* 269–308.

Cocude, M., Mellet, E., & Denis, M. (1999). Visual and mental exploration of visuo-spatial configurations: Behavioral and neuroimaging approaches. *Psychological Research, 62,* 93–106.

Cranberg, L. D., & Albert, M. L. (1988). Chess mind. In L. Obler & D. Fein (Eds.), *The exceptional brain: Neuropsychology of talent and special abilities* (pp. 156–190). New York: Guilford.

De Groot, A. D. (1965). *Thought and choice in chess.* The Hague, The Netherlands: Mouton.

De Groot, A. D. (1966). Perception and memory versus thought: Some old ideas and recent findings. In B. Kleinmuntz (Ed.), *Problem solving* (pp. 19–50). New York: Wiley.

De Groot, A. D., & Gobet, F. (1996). *Perception and memory in chess.* Assen, The Netherlands: van Gorcum.

Djakov, I. N., Petrovsky, N. B., & Rudik, P. A. (1926). *Psihologia shakhmatnoi igry* [Chess psychology]. Moscow: Avtorov.

Elo, A. E. (1978). *The ratings of chess players: Past and present.* London: Batsford.

Ericsson, K. A., & Kintsch, W. (1995). Long-term working memory. *Psychological Review, 102,* 211–245.

Farah, M. J. (1985). Psychophysical evidence for a shared representational medium for mental images and percepts. *Journal of Experimental Psychology: General, 114,* 92–103.

Fiez, J. A. (2001). Bridging the gap between neuroimaging and neuropsychology: Challenges and potential benefits. *Journal of Clinical and Experimental Neuropsychiatry, 23,* 19–31.

Finke, R. A. (1985). Theories relating mental imagery to perception. *Psychological Bulletin, 98,* 236–256.

Frey, P. W., & Adesman, P. (1976). Recall memory for visually presented chess positions. *Memory and Cognition, 4,* 541–547.

Friston, K. J., Ashburner, J., Frith, C., Poline, J.-B., Heather, J., & Frackowiak, R. (1995a). Spatial registration and normalization of images. *Human Brain Mapping, 2,* 165–189.

Friston, K. J., Holmes, A., Worsley, K., Poline, J.-B., Frith, C., & Frackowiak, R. (1995b). Statistical parametric mapping in functional imaging: A general linear approach. *Human Brain Mapping, 2,* 189–210.

Gobet, F. (1998). Expert memory: Comparison of four theories. *Cognition, 66,* 115–152.

Gobet, F., & Simon, H. A. (1996). Templates in chess memory: A mechanism for recalling several boards. *Cognitive Psychology, 31,* 1–40.

Holding, D. H. (1985). *The psychology of chess skill.* Hillsdale, NJ: Lawrence Erlbaum Associates, Inc.

Holm, S., Law, I., & Paulson, O. (1996). 3D PET activation studies with H2150 bolus injection: Count rate performance and dose optimization. In D. Bailey, V. Cunningham, T. Jones, & R. Myers (Eds.), *Quantification of brain function using PET.* San Diego: Academic Press.

Just, M. A., Carpenter, P. A., Maguire, M., Diwadkar, V., & McMains, S. (2001). Mental rotation of objects retrieved from memory: A functional MRI study of spatial processing. *Journal of Experimental Psychology: General, 130,* 493–504.

Kant, I. (1787). *Kritik der reinen Vernunft* [The critique of pure reason]. Stuttgart, Germany: Philip Reclam.

Kosslyn, S. M. (1980). *Image and mind.* Cambridge, MA: Harvard University Press.

Kosslyn, S. M. (1994). *Image and brain: The resolution of the imagery debate.* Cambridge, MA: MIT Press.

Krogius, N. (1976). *Psychology in chess.* New York: RHM Press.

Laine, M., Rinne, J. O., Krause, B. J., Teräs, M., & Sipilä, H. (1999). Left hemisphere activation during processing of morphologically complex word forms in adults. *Neuroscience Letters, 271,* 85–88.

Leibniz, G. (1979). *New essays on human understanding.* Cambridge, UK: Cambridge University Press. (Original work published 1704.)

Lewellen, T., Kohlmyer, S., Miyaoka, R., Kaplan, M., Stearns, C., & Schubert, S. (1996). Investigation of the performance of the General Electric ADVANCE Positron Emission Tomograph in 3D Mode. *IEEE Transactions on Nuclear Science, 43,* 2199–2206.

Mellet, E., Tzourio-Mazoyer, N., Bricogne, S., Mazoyer, B., Kosslyn, S. M., & Denis, M. (2000). Functional anatomy of high-resolution visual mental imagery. *Journal of Cognitive Neuroscience, 12,* 98–109.

Milojkovic, J. (1982). Chess imagery in novice and master. *Journal of Mental Imagery, 6,* 125–144.

Moscovitch, M., Behrmann, M., & Winocur, G. (1994). Do PETS have long or short ears? Mental imagery and neuroimaging. *Trends in Neurosciences, 17,* 292–294.

Newell, A., & Simon, H. A. (1972). *Human problem solving.* Englewood Cliffs, NJ: Prentice-Hall.

Nichelli, P., Grafman, J., Pietrini, P., Alway, D., Carton, J. C., & Miletich, R. (1994). Brain activity in chess playing. *Nature, 369,* 191.

Robbins, T. W., Anderson, E., Barker, D. R., Bradley, A. C., Fearnyhough, R., Henson, R., Hudson, S. R., & Baddeley, A. D. (1995). Working memory in chess. *Memory and Cognition, 24,* 83–93.

Saariluoma, P. (1985). Chess players' intake of task relevant cues. *Memory and Cognition, 13,* 385–391.

Saariluoma, P. (1989). Chess players' recall of auditorily presented chess positions. *European Journal of Cognitive Psychology, 1,* 309–320.

Saariluoma, P. (1990). Apperception and restructuring in chess players' problem solving. In K. J. Gilhooly, M. T. G. Keane, R. H. Logie, & G. Erdos (Eds.), *Lines of thought: Reflections on the psychology of thinking* (pp. 41–57). Wiley: London.

Saariluoma, P. (1991). Aspects of skilled imagery in blindfold chess. *Acta Psychologica, 77,* 65–89.

Saariluoma, P. (1992a). Do visual images have gestalt properties? *Quarterly Journal of Experimental Psychology, 45A,* 399–420.

Saariluoma, P. (1992b). Error in chess: Apperception restructuring view. *Psychological Research, 54,* 17–26.

Saariluoma, P. (1992c). Visuo-spatial and articulatory interference in chess players' information intake. *Applied Cognitive Psychology, 6,* 77–89.

Saariluoma, P. (1994). Location coding in chess. *Quarterly Journal of Experimental Psychology, 47A,* 607–630.

Saariluoma, P. (1995). *Chess players' thinking.* London: Routledge.

Saariluoma, P. (1997). *Foundational analysis.* London: Routledge.

Saariluoma, P. (1998). Adversary problem-solving and working memory. In R. H. Logie & K. H. Gilhooly (Eds.), *Working memory and thinking.* Hove, UK: Psychology Press.

Saariluoma, P. (2001). Chess and content-oriented psychology of thinking. *Psicologica, 22,* 143–164.

Saariluoma, P., & Kalakoski, V. (1997). Skilled imagery and long-term working memory. *American Journal of Psychology, 110,* 177–201.

Saariluoma, P., & Kalakoski, V. (1998). Apperception and imagery in blindfold chess. *Memory, 6,* 67–90.

Shallice, T. (2002). Fractionation of the supervisory system. In D. Stuss & R. Knight (Eds.), *Principles of frontal lobe functions* (pp. 261–277). Oxford, UK: Oxford University Press.

Stout, G. F. (1896). *Analytic psychology.* New York: Macmillan.

Talairach, J., & Tournoux, P. (1988). *Co-planar stereotaxic atlas of the human brain.* Stuttgart, Germany: Thieme.

Vicente, K. J. (1988). Adapting the memory recall paradigm to evaluate interfaces. *Acta Psychologica, 69,* 249–278.

Vicente, K. J., & de Groot, A. D. (1990). The memory recall paradigm: Straightening out the historical record. *American Psychologist, 45,* 285–287.

Wundt, W. (1880). *Logik.* Stuttgart, Germany: Ferdinand Enke.

Subject index